D0341176

THE LITTLE BOOK OF
HYGGE

THE LITTLE BOOK OF
HYGGE

Danish Secrets to
Happy Living

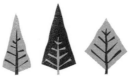

MEIK WIKING

WM

WILLIAM MORROW
An Imprint of HarperCollins *Publishers*

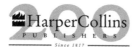

THE LITTLE BOOK OF HYGGE. Copyright © 2017 by Meik Wiking. All rights reserved. Printed in Bosnia and Herzegovina. No part of this book may be used or reproduced in any manner whatsoever without written permission except in the case of brief quotations embodied in critical articles and reviews. For information address HarperCollins Publishers, 195 Broadway, New York, NY 10007.

HarperCollins books may be purchased for educational, business, or sales promotional use. For information please e-mail the Special Markets Department at SPsales@harpercollins.com.

Originally published in the United Kingdom in 2016 by Penguin Random House UK.

Lyrics on page 178 from "The Happy Day of Svante" by Benny Andersen are from Hojskolesangbogen, translated by Kurt Hansen

Designed by Hampton Associates

Library of Congress Cataloging-in-Publication Data has been applied for.

ISBN 978-0-06-265880-7

23 24 GPS 20 19

CONTENTS

INTRODUCTION vi

THE KEY TO HAPPINESS? viii

LIGHT 1

WE NEED TO TALK ABOUT HYGGE 15

TOGETHERNESS 33

FOOD AND DRINK 51

CLOTHING 81

HOME 89

HYGGE OUTSIDE THE HOME 111

HYGGE ALL YEAR ROUND 123

HYGGE ON THE CHEAP 137

HYGGE TOUR OF COPENHAGEN 155

CHRISTMAS 161

SUMMER HYGGE 183

FIVE DIMENSIONS OF HYGGE 195

HYGGE AND HAPPINESS 205

INTRODUCTION

Hooga? Hhyooguh? Heurgh? It is not important how you choose to pronounce or even spell hygge. *To paraphrase one of the greatest philosophers of our time—Winnie-the-Pooh—when asked how to spell a certain emotion, "You don't spell it, you feel it."*

However, spelling and pronouncing *hygge* is the easy part. Explaining exactly what it is, that's the tricky part. Hygge has been called everything from "the art of creating intimacy," "coziness of the soul," and "the absence of annoyance," to "taking pleasure from the presence of soothing things," "cozy togetherness," and my personal favorite, "cocoa by candlelight".

Hygge is about an atmosphere and an experience, rather than about things. It is about being with the people we love. A feeling of home. A feeling that we are safe, that we are shielded from the world and allow ourselves to let our guard down. You may be having an endless conversation about the small or big things in life—or just be comfortable in each other's silent company—or simply just be by yourself enjoying a cup of tea.

One December just before Christmas, I was spending the weekend with some friends at an old cabin. The shortest day of the year was brightened by the blanket of snow covering the surrounding landscape. When the sun set, around four in the afternoon, we would not see it again for seventeen hours, and we headed inside to get the fire going.

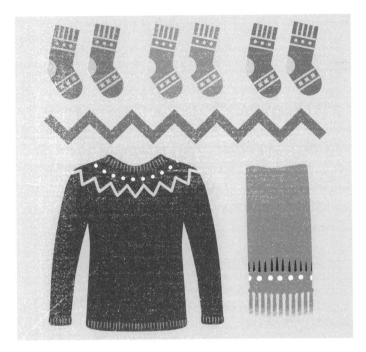

We were all tired after hiking and were half asleep, sitting in a semicircle around the fireplace in the cabin, wearing big sweaters and woolen socks. The only sounds you could hear were the stew boiling, the sparks from the fireplace, and someone having a sip of mulled wine. Then one of my friends broke the silence.

"Could this be any more hygge?" he asked rhetorically.

"Yes," one of the women said after a moment. "If there was a storm raging outside."

We all nodded.

THE KEY TO HAPPINESS?

I have the best job in the world. I study what makes people happy. At the Happiness Research Institute, which is an independent think tank focusing on well-being, happiness, and quality of life, we explore the causes and effects of human happiness and work toward improving the quality of life of citizens across the world.

We are based in Denmark, and yes, we do have lit candles at the office Monday to Friday, and yes, our office was partly chosen because of the hygge factor. No fireplace, though. Yet. But we were also founded and are based in Denmark because the country consistently ranks among the happiest nations in the world. Denmark is by no means a perfect utopia, and the country faces challenges and issues like any other country, but I do believe Denmark can be a source of inspiration for how countries can increase the quality of life of their citizens.

Denmark's position as one of the happiest countries in the world has created a lot of media interest. On a weekly basis, I am asked questions like "Why are the Danes so happy?" and "What can we learn from the Danes when it comes to happiness?" from journalists from _The New York Times_, the BBC, _The Guardian_, the _China Daily_, and _The Washington Post_, among others. In addition, delegations of mayors, researchers, and policy makers from all corners of the earth frequently visit the Happiness Research Institute in pursuit of . . . well . . . happiness—or at least in pursuit of the reasons for the high levels of happiness, well-being, and quality of life people enjoy in

Denmark. To many, it is quite the mystery, as besides the horrific weather, Danes are also subject to some of the highest tax rates in the world.

Interestingly, there is wide support for the welfare state. The support stems from an awareness of the fact that the welfare model turns our collective wealth into well-being. We are not paying taxes, we are investing in our society. We are purchasing quality of life. The key to understanding the high levels of well-being in Denmark is the welfare model's ability to reduce risk, uncertainty, and anxiety among its citizens and to prevent extreme unhappiness.

However, recently, I have also come to realize that there might be an overlooked ingredient in the Danish recipe for happiness— hygge. The word *hygge* originates from a Norwegian word meaning "well-being". For almost five hundred years, Denmark and Norway were one kingdom, until Denmark lost Norway in 1814. *Hygge* appeared in written Danish for the first time in the early 1800s, and the link between hygge and well-being or happiness may be no coincidence.

Danes are the happiest people in Europe according to the European Social Survey, but they are also the ones who meet most often with their friends and family and feel the calmest and most peaceful. Therefore, it is with good reason that we see a growing interest in hygge. Journalists are touring Denmark searching for hygge; in the UK, a college is now teaching Danish hygge; and around the world, hygge bakeries, shops, and cafés are popping up. But how do you create hygge? How are hygge and happiness linked? And what is hygge exactly? Those are some of the questions this book seeks to answer.

THE LITTLE BOOK OF
HYGGE

CHAPTER ONE

—

LIGHT

INSTANT HYGGE: CANDLES

No recipe for hygge is complete without candles. When Danes are asked what they most associate with hygge, an overwhelming 85 percent will mention candles.

The word for "spoilsport" in Danish is *lyseslukker*, which means "the one who puts out the candles", and this is no coincidence. There is no faster way to get to hygge than to light a few candles or, as they are called in Danish, *levende lys*, or living lights. The American ambassador to Denmark, Rufus Gifford, said of the Danes' love affair with candles: "I mean, it is not just in the living room. It is everywhere. In your classrooms, in your boardrooms. As an American, you think, 'Fire hazard!—how can you possibly have an open flame in your classroom?' It is kind of an emotional happiness, an emotional coziness."

The American ambassador is onto something. According to the European Candle Association, Denmark burns more candles per head than anywhere in Europe. Each Dane burns around thirteen pounds of candle wax each year. To put this in context, each Dane consumes around six and a half pounds of bacon per year (yes, bacon consumption per capita is a standard metric in Denmark). The candle consumption is a European record. In fact, Denmark burns almost twice as much candle wax as the runner-up, Austria, with a little under seven pounds per year. However, scented candles are not a big thing. In fact, Asp-Holmblad, Denmark's oldest producer of candles, doesn't even include scented candles in their product range. Scented candles are considered artificial, and Danes prefer natural and organic products. In fact, Danes rank towards the top of the list in Europe when it comes to buying organic.

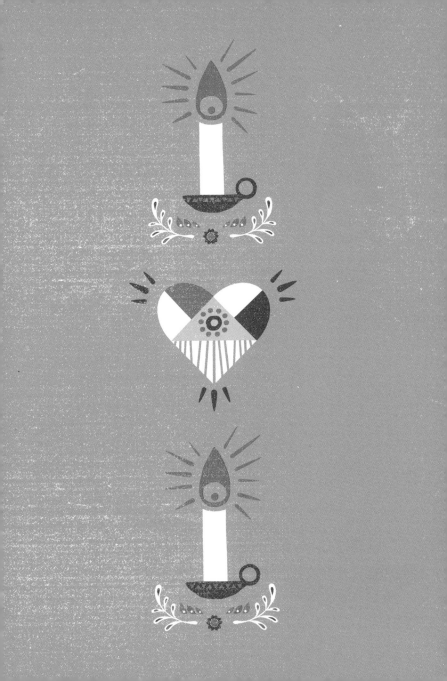

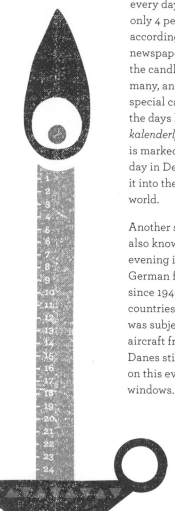

More than half of Danes light candles almost every day during autumn and winter, and only 4 percent say they never light candles, according to a survey by one of the major newspapers in Denmark. During December, the candle consumption soars to thrice as many, and this is also the time to witness the special candle that is to be burned only in the days leading up to Christmas, namely the *kalenderlys*—the advent candle. This candle is marked with twenty-four lines, one for each day in December before Christmas, turning it into the slowest countdown clock in the world.

Another special candle occasion is May 4, also known as *lysfest*, or light party. On this evening in 1945, the BBC broadcast that the German forces who had occupied Denmark since 1940 had surrendered. As in many countries during World War II, Denmark was subject to blackouts to prevent enemy aircraft from navigating by city lights. Today, Danes still celebrate the return of the light on this evening by putting candles in their windows.

Hyggelige as the Danes may be, there is one serious drawback to being crazy about candles: the soot. Studies show that lighting just one candle fills the air with more microparticles than traffic in a busy street.

A study undertaken by the Danish Building Research Institute showed that candles shed more particles indoors than either cigarettes or cooking. Despite Denmark being a highly regulated country, we have yet to see warning labels on candles. Nobody messes with the hygge fanatics. There is now a growing awareness among Danes of the importance of airing out a room after burning candles. Nevertheless, despite the health implications, Danes continue to consume candles in obscene quantities.

How often do Danes light candles?

28%	23%	23%	8%	4%	14%
Every day	4–6 days per week	1–3 days per week	Less than 1–3 days per month	Never	Don't know

How many candles are lit at a time?

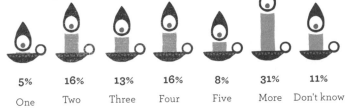

5%	16%	13%	16%	8%	31%	11%
One	Two	Three	Four	Five	More	Don't know

LAMPS

Lighting is not just about candles. Danes are obsessed by lighting in general. I once spent two hours walking around Rome with my girlfriend at the time to find a restaurant that had hyggelig *lighting.*

Danes select lamps carefully and place them strategically to create soothing pools of light. It is an art form, a science, and an industry. Some of the most beautifully designed lamps in the world come from the golden age of Danish design—for example, the lamps of Poul Henningsen, Arne Jacobsen, and Verner Panton. Visit a student on a shoestring budget and you may still encounter a $1,300 Verner Panton lamp in the corner of her hundred-square-foot flat.

The rule of thumb is: the lower the temperature of the light, the more hygge. A camera flash is around 5,500 Kelvin (K), fluorescent tubes are 5,000K, incandescent lamps 3,000K, while sunsets and wood and candle flames are about 1,800K. That is your hygge sweet spot.

The closest you will ever come to seeing vampires burned by daylight is by inviting a group of Danes for a hygge dinner and then placing them under a 5,000K fluorescent light tube. At first they will squint, trying to examine the torture device you have placed in the ceiling. Then, as dinner begins, observe how they move uncomfortably around in their chairs, compulsively scratching and trying to suppress twitches.

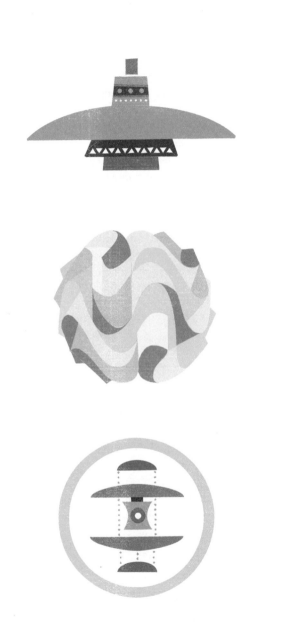

The obsession with lighting comes from the lack of contact with it in the natural world from October to March. During this time, the only resource Denmark has in abundance is darkness. Summers in Denmark are beautiful. When the first rays of light reach the country, Danes awaken from their hibernation and fall over themselves to find spots in the sun. I love summer in Denmark. It is my favorite time of the year. And if it wasn't bad enough that winters are dark and cold and summers are short, Denmark also has 179 days of rain per year. *Game of Thrones* fans, think of the city of Winterfell.

That is why hygge has been refined to the level it has, and why it is seen as part of the national identity and culture in Denmark. Hygge is the antidote to the cold winter, the rainy days, and the duvet of darkness. So while you can have hygge all year round, it is during winter that it becomes not only a necessity but a survival strategy. That is why Danes have a reputation of being hygge fundamentalists and talk about it ... a lot.

My favorite spot in my apartment in Copenhagen is the windowsill in the kitchen-dining area. It is wide enough to sit comfortably in and I've added pillows and blankets to make it a real *hyggekrog* (see the hygge dictionary on page 26). The radiator underneath the windowsill makes it the perfect place to enjoy a cup of tea on a cold winter night. But what I like about it most is the warm amber glow issuing from every apartment across the courtyard. It's a constantly changing mosaic of radiance as people leave and return home. In part, I owe this view to Poul Henningsen. Inevitably, a well-lit room in Denmark is likely to hold a lamp by the architect and designer all Danes know simply as PH.

He was to light fixtures what Edison was to the lightbulb. PH was, like most Danes today, obsessed with light. Some call him the world's first lighting architect, as he devoted his career to exploring the importance of light for our well-being, aiming to develop a lamp that could spread light without subjecting people to a direct glare.

Poul Henningsen was born in 1894 and did not grow up with electric light but in the soft glow of petroleum lamps. These were his source of inspiration. His designs shape and refine the power of the electric light yet maintain the softness of the light of a petroleum lamp.

> *It doesn't cost money to light a room correctly—but it does require culture. From the age of eighteen, when I began to experiment with light, I have been searching for harmony in lighting. Human beings are like children. As soon as they get new toys, they throw away their culture and the orgy starts. The electric light gave the possibility of wallowing in light.*
>
> *When, in the evening, from the top of a tram car, you look into all the homes on the first floor, you shudder at how dismal people's homes are. Furniture, style, carpets—everything in the home is unimportant, compared to the positioning of the lighting.*
>
> **Poul Henningsen** *(1894–1967), "On Light"*

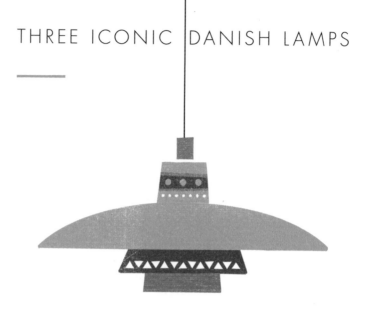

 ## THE PH LAMP

After a decade of experiments with lamps and lighting in
his attic, Henningsen presented the first PH lamp in 1925.
It gave a softer and more diffused light by using a series of
layered shades to disperse the light yet conceal the lightbulb.
In addition, to bring the harsh white light toward the red end
of the spectrum, PH gave the inner side of one element of the
shade a red colour. His biggest success was PH5, which has
metal shades and was launched in 1958, but PH lamps have
now been produced in over a thousand different designs.
Many of these are not in production anymore, and the rarest
lamps can go for more than $25,000 at auction.

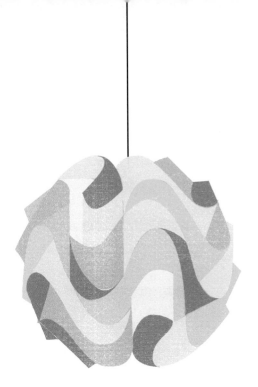

 LE KLINT

In 1943, the Klint family started producing lampshades with folding pleats, but in fact they had been designed four decades earlier by Peder Vilhelm Jensen-Klint, a Danish architect, for his own use, as he had designed a petroleum lamp and needed a shade. It became a family business, applying the skills in design, innovation, and business of the sons and daughters of Klint.

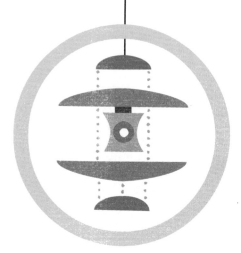

③ PANTON VP GLOBE

The Panton VP Globe is a pendant lamp that casts calming,
diffused light from its center rim. It was designed in 1969
by Verner Panton—the *enfant terrible* of Danish design who
loved to work with modern materials such as plastic and steel.
Panton attended the Royal Danish Academy of Fine Arts,
Schools of Architecture, Design and Conservation, a leading
institution for architecture, which today includes a "light
laboratory" that examines daylight and artificial lighting.

BETTER THAN PHOTOSHOP

Members of one profession might be just as obsessed with lighting as the Danes: photographers. Photography means painting with light, and doing it increases your understanding of light and your ability to see and appreciate it.

This might be the reason why I love photography and have taken tens of thousands of pictures over the past ten years, and why my favorite light is the golden hour. The golden hour is roughly the first hour after sunrise and the last hour before sunset. When the sun is low in the sky, the sunlight has to travel through a greater depth of atmosphere. During these times, it produces a warm, soft, diffused light. It is sometimes also called the "magic hour", and I think I have fallen in love with every woman whose picture I have taken at this time of day for that 1/250 of a second. This is the light you want to aim for if you are going for *hyggelig* lighting indoors. The flattering quality of the lighting will make you and all your friends look "grotto-fabulous." It's better than any Instagram filter.

> **HYGGE TIP:** CREATE *HYGGELIG* LIGHTING
>
> You guessed it. Bring out the candles. But remember to air out the room. However, you may also want to consider your electric-light strategy. Usually, several smaller lamps around the room create a more *hyggeligt* light than one big lamp set in the ceiling. You want to create small caves of light around the room.

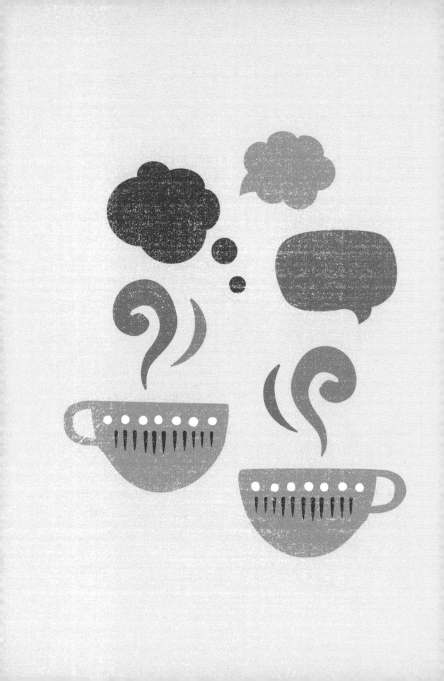

CHAPTER TWO

WE NEED TO
TALK ABOUT
HYGGE

IT'S ALL ABOUT THE HYGGE

The Danish language has been called many things, but seldom beautiful. Google "Danish sounds like . . . ," and the first two suggestions that appear are "German" and "potato." To foreigners, Danish sounds like someone speaking German with a hot potato in their mouth.

To be fair, some people have also suggested it sounds somewhat like a diseased seal choking. Nevertheless, it is rich when it comes to describing hygge.

Hygge comes in the form of both a verb and an adjective. Something can be *hyggelig(t)* (hygge-like): What a *hyggelig* living room! It was so *hyggeligt* to see you! Have a *hyggelig* time!

We throw the words *hygge* and *hyggelig* around so much that, to foreigners, it might appear excessive. We have to state how *hyggelig* everything is. All the time. And not just in the hygge moment itself. We talk about how *hyggeligt* it will be to get together on Friday, and on Monday we will remind each other of how *hyggelig* Friday was.

Hygge is a key performance indicator of most Danish social gatherings. "Honey, do you think our guests *hyggede* themselves?" (It's the past tense—don't attempt to pronounce it.)

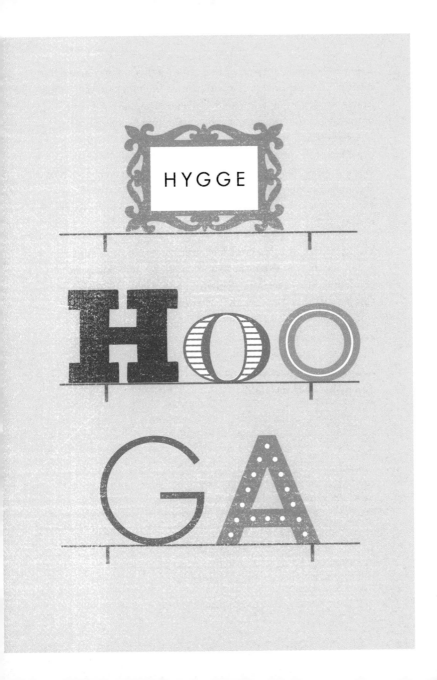

HYGGE

HOO

GA

Every few weeks, I meet up with a group of guys to play poker. It is quite an international group, with people from Mexico, the United States, Turkey, France, England, India and Denmark. Over the years, we have covered most subjects ranging from women to how to optimize the range of an orange cannon. Due to the diversity of the group, our conversations are always in English. Nevertheless, there is one Danish word that is often used around the table. You guessed it. Often it will come from Danny from Mexico after losing a big hand: "It doesn't matter. I am just here for the hygge."

The hygge factor is not just a key performance indicator for social events, it is also a not so unique selling point for cafés and restaurants. Search for "beautiful restaurant" in Danish, and Google will provide you with 7,000 hits. Searching for a "quality restaurant" will give you 9,600 options and "cheap restaurant," 30,600. "*Hyggelig* restaurant" gives you 88,900 hits on Google. As Lonely Planet points out, "The Danes are obsessed with

Can hygge be translated?

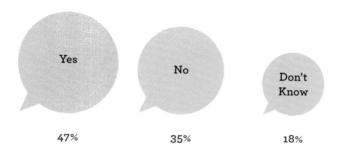

Yes 47%

No 35%

Don't Know 18%

coziness. All of them. Even the toughest leather-clad biker will recommend a bar based on its 'hygge' factor."

It means that everything you learned in that marketing class was wrong. Price, product, place, and promotion can kiss my ass. It is all about the hygge. I live in Copenhagen. Cafés are plentiful, and there is one right across the street from my apartment. Their coffee is an abomination. It tastes like *fish* (yes, I was surprised too) and costs five euros. I still go there sometimes. They have an open fireplace, so it's hygge.

Fireplaces are not unique to Denmark. Neither are candles, cozy company or snuggling up with a cup of tea and a blanket on a stormy night. Danes, however, insist that hygge is uniquely Danish. One third refuse the idea that hygge can be translated into other languages and believe that it is mainly practiced in Denmark.

Is hygge mainly practiced in Denmark?

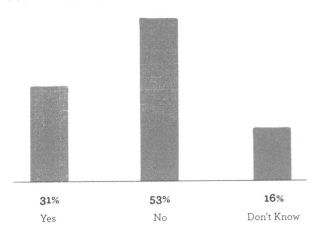

31%	**53%**	**16%**
Yes	No	Don't Know

Source: the Happiness Research Institute

I disagree with that. Danes are not the only ones who can have hygge or identify it, and other languages have similar expressions. The Dutch call it *gezelligheid* and Germans talk of *Gemütlichkeit*, a sense of well-being based on good food and good company, and Canadians will recognize it as "hominess." However, while more languages than Danish have similar adjectives for the noun *hygge*, it seems that only Danes use *hygge* as a verb, as in "Why don't you come over and hygge with us tonight?" This might be unique.

What might also be unique for Denmark when it comes to hygge is how much we talk about it, focus on it, and consider it as a defining feature of our cultural identity and an integral part of the national DNA. In other words, what freedom is to Americans, thoroughness to Germans, and the stiff upper lip to the British, hygge is to Danes.

Because of its importance to Danish culture and identity, the Danish language is also rich when it comes to talking about hygge.

Danish is an infinite list of compound words. For example, *speciallægepraksisplanlægningsstabiliseringsperiode* (specialty-doctor-practice-planning-stabilizing-period) is an actual word. It contains fifty-one letters and could be considered the golden goal of Scrabble.

Hygge is no different. You can pretty much add it to any other word in the Danish language. You can be a *hyggespreder* (someone who spreads the hygge), Friday night is reserved for *familiehygge*, and socks can be labeled *hyggesokker.* At the Happiness Research Institute, we have a sign saying:

|| *"You are welcome to borrow some woolen* hyggesokker *if your feet are cold."*

WHAT'S IN A NAME?

Shakespeare famously wrote, in Romeo and Juliet, *"What's in a name? That which we call a rose/By any other name would smell as sweet," and I think his point applies to hygge as well.*

Danes are not the only ones who can enjoy the atmosphere, comfort, and pleasure that comes from being in good company, in front of the fire, with some mulled wine.

While an English translation of *hygge* as coziness may be problematic, because it loses a lot of important associations, we can find a variety of concepts more similar to hygge around the world.

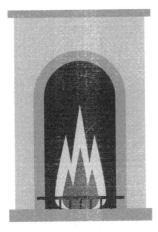
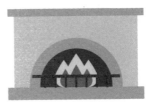

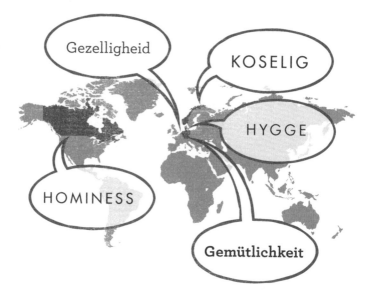

GEZELLIGHEID—THE NETHERLANDS

Dictionaries tell us that *gezelligheid* is something cozy, quaint, or nice, but to the Dutch, *gezelligheid* goes way beyond this.

If you want to score some cheap points with the Dutch, go with what President Obama stated when he visited the Netherlands in 2014: "I'm told there's a Dutch word that captures the spirit, which doesn't translate exactly in English, but let me say that my first visit to the Netherlands has been truly *gezellig*."

The Dutch tend to use the word *gezellig* in a lot of ways—for example, drinking coffee at a *gezellig* café (read: warm interior, flickering candles, and a sleeping cat). Seeking shelter from the pouring rain at a *gezellig* bar that serves only vintage beers and plays old records is the purest form of *gezelligheid*. Sitting in a soulless waiting room for your appointment with the dentist is everything but *gezellig*, unless a very *gezellig* friend accompanies you. Are you starting to see the similarities between *gezelligheid* and hygge?

Even though the two are very similar, they are not completely alike, and it's often emphasized that *gezelligheid* is a bit more social than hygge. To test whether this is the case, we carried out a small survey among Dutch people, and the results seem to back up this theory.

On most of the indicators, it seems that Danes experience hygge the same way the Dutch experience *gezelligheid*. The concept is important in both cultures, and candles, fireplaces, and Christmas are core elements in hygge and *gezelligheid*. However, the notion that *gezelligheid* has a more outgoing dimension than hygge is also supported by the data we collected. The majority of Dutch people (57 percent) agree that you experience the most *gezelligheid* outside of your home, while only 27 percent of Danes find that it's most *hyggeligt* to go out. In addition, 62 percent of the Dutch agree that summer is the most *gezellig* season of the year, while Danes prefer autumn in terms of hygge.

KOSELIG — NORWAY

For Norwegians, everything should, ideally, be *koselig*. Yet again, do not mistake this word for "coziness" (say the Norwegians).

More than anything, *koselig* is a feeling of warmth, intimacy, and getting together. A perfect *koselig* evening would consist of good food on the table, warm colors around you, a group of good friends, and a fireplace, or at least some lighted candles.

HOMINESS—CANADA

Canadians use the word *hominess* to describe a state of shutting out the outside world. It implies a feeling of community, warmth, and togetherness, but hominess also refers to things that resemble home or echo the feeling of home. Thus it has both a physical and a symbolic dimension: it describes how property can be homey if it's authentic and "real" and how a situation can be homey if it somehow brings to mind the state or feeling of seeking shelter and shutting out the outside world. So, just like *hygge*, hominess very much implies a feeling of authenticity, warmth, and togetherness.

GEMÜTLICHKEIT—GERMANY

Germans use the word *Gemütlichkeit* to cover the state of warmth, friendliness, and belonging, and often to describe the atmosphere at a German beer garden. Visiting an Oktoberfest in Germany, you are even likely to hear the song *"Ein Prost der Gemütlichkeit"* ("A Toast to Coziness").

Which season is most *hyggelig/gezellig*?

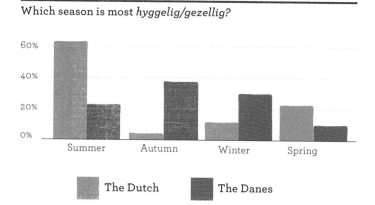

HYGGE IS FOR EVERYONE

The list of concepts above doesn't only provide evidence that it is possible for people other than Danes to experience hygge but also that they already do.

While the concepts across countries aren't completely identical, what they all share is that they are more developed and complex versions of a feeling of coziness, warmth, and togetherness. The various words denote groups of different activities and settings that generate similar and related feelings, which have merged into linguistic concepts.

Danish hygge and Dutch *gezelligheid* may stand out a bit from the others, though, as they are so integrated in daily conversation and lifestyle. But one could ask whether this is in any way beneficial. It may be difficult to provide a simple answer to this question. But it is worth mentioning that, according to the European Social Survey, Denmark and the Netherlands are among the countries with the fewest people who seldom enjoy life or rarely feel calm and relaxed. Also, these two countries represent the very top of the official happiness charts commissioned by the UN.

So what's in a name? On the one hand, the specific name has no value in itself. Hygge works just as well as hominess or *gezelligheid*. On the other hand, we use names to capture that feeling of coziness, warmth, and togetherness, to shape it into a more fixed concept, and eventually, we develop a phenomenon that marks our unique cultural traits. Throughout this book, I will point toward things, experiences, and moments that are hygge so you will come to an understanding of exactly what hygge is.

HYGGE DICTIONARY

___

Our words shape our actions. So here are some new words that will help you get your hygge on.

Fredagshygge/Søndagshygge *[Fredashooga/Sundashooga]*

Hygge you have on Fridays or Sundays. After a long week, *fredagshygge* usually means the family curling up on the couch together watching TV. *Søndagshygge* is about having a slow day with tea, books, music, blankets, and perhaps the occasional walk if things go crazy.

> "A fredagshygge *tradition in the family was candy and watching a Disney movie.*"

Hyggebukser *[hoogabucksr]*

That one pair of pants you would never wear in public but are so comfortable that they are likely to be, secretly, your favorites.

> "*She just needed a day for herself, so she stayed at home in her* hyggebukser, *wore no makeup, and just watched television all day.*"

Hyggehjørnet *[hoogajornet]*

To be in the mood for hygge. Literal meaning: "the corner of hygge."

> "*I am in* hyggehjørnet."

Hyggekrog *[hoogacrow]*

The nook of a kitchen or living room where one can sit and have a *hyggelig* time.

> "*Let's sit in the* hyggekrog."

Hyggeonkel *[hoogaunkel]*

A person who plays with the kids and may be a little too lenient. Literal meaning: "the uncle of hygge."

❚❚ *"He is such a* hyggeonkel.*"*

Hyggesnak *[hoogasnak]*

Chitchat or cozy conversation that doesn't touch on controversial issues.

❚❚ *"We* hyggesnakkede *for a couple of hours."*

Hyggestund *[hoogastun]*

A moment of hygge.

❚❚ *"He poured himself a cup of coffee and sat in his window for a* hyggestund.*"*

Uhyggeligt *[uh-hoogalit]*

While hygge and *hyggelig* may be difficult to translate into English, it is not the case when it comes to the antonym of hygge. *Uhyggeligt* (un-hygge) means "creepy" or "scary," and this provides us with some insight into how central the feeling of safety is to hygge.

❚❚ *"Walking alone through the woods at night is* uhyggeligt *if you hear a wolf howling."*

As my friend pointed out in the cabin in Sweden, the evening would have been even more hygge if there had been a storm outside. Perhaps hygge is even more hygge if there is a controlled element of danger—of *uhygge*. A storm, thunder, or a scary movie.

WHERE DOES HYGGE COME FROM?

Hygge appeared in written Danish for the first time in the early 1800s, but the word is actually Norwegian in origin.

Between 1397 and 1814, Denmark and Norway were one kingdom. Danes and Norwegians still understand each other's languages today.

The original word in Norwegian means well-being. However, _hygge_ might originate from the word _hug_. _Hug_ comes from the 1560s word _hugge_, which means "to embrace." The word _hugge_ is of unknown origin—maybe it originates from the Old Norse _hygga_, which means "to comfort," which comes from the word _hugr_, meaning "mood." In turn, that word comes from the Germanic word _hugjan_, which relates to the Old English _hycgan_, meaning "to think, consider." Interestingly, _consideration_, _mood_, _comfort_, _hug_ and _well-being_ may all be words to describe elements of what hygge is today.

HYGGE TIP: GET YOUR DANISH ON

Start throwing those hygge words around. Invite your friends for a _hyggelig_ evening and create compound words like there is no tomorrow. You may also want to put the hygge manifesto on your fridge to remind you to hygge every day.

A GLOBAL CONVERSATION ABOUT HYGGE

Hygge seems to be the talk of the town these days.

"Hygge: A heart-warming lesson from Denmark" writes the BBC; "Get cozy: why we should all embrace the Danish art of 'hygge.'" says *The Telegraph*; and Morley College in London is now teaching students how to hygge. The Hygge Bakery in Los Angeles is providing Danish *romkugler* [rum-cool-r] (rum balls), rum-flavored chocolate treats, originally made by Danish bakers to use up left-over pastry. In the book *The Danish Way of Parenting*, you can find extensive chapters on how hygge is the way to raise the happiest children in the world.

THE HYGGE MANIFESTO

---

1. ATMOSPHERE

Turn down the lights.

2. PRESENCE

Be here now. Turn off the phones.

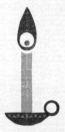

3. PLEASURE

Coffee, chocolate, cookies, cakes, candy. Gimme! Gimme! Gimme!

4. EQUALITY

"We" over "me." Share the tasks and the airtime.

5. GRATITUDE

Take it in. This might be as good as it gets.

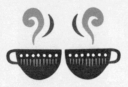

6. HARMONY

It's not a competition. We already like you. There is no need to brag about your achievements.

7. COMFORT

Get comfy. Take a break. It's all about relaxation.

8. TRUCE

No drama. Let's discuss politics another day.

9. TOGETHERNESS

Build relationships and narratives. "Do you remember the time we ... ?"

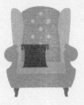

10. SHELTER

This is your tribe. This is a place of peace and security.

CHAPTER THREE

————

TOGETHERNESS

LIKE A HUG
WITHOUT TOUCHING

———

Every year, my friends and I go skiing in the Alps (the last time, someone even packed candles). We all enjoy the speed, the thrill, the flow, and the exercise of the slopes, but to me, the best part of the day is the hour after we come back to our cabin.

Your feet ache, your body is used and tired, you find a chair on the balcony, and the distinct sound of Grand Marnier being poured tells you that coffee is ready. More people come to the balcony, you are all still wearing your ski clothes, too tired to change, too tired to talk, too tired for anything but to enjoy one another's silent company, take in the view, and breathe in the air of the mountain.

When I give lectures about happiness research, I ask the audience to close their eyes and tell them to think of the last time they felt really happy. Sometimes people become a little uneasy, but I assure them that I am not going to ask them to share their memory with the rest of the class. You can almost pinpoint the moment when people have their happy memory in their mind, as peaceful smiles light up the room. When I ask people to raise their hand if they were with others in their memories, usually nine out of ten do so.

Of course, this is not a scientific method and therefore proves nothing, but it does allow people to attach a memory and an emotion to the dry statistics I then launch at them. The reason why I want them to remember this is that, in all the work I have done within the field of happiness research, this is the point I am surest about: the best predictor of whether we are happy or not is our social relationships. It is the clearest and most recurrent pattern I see when I look at the evidence on why some people are happier than others.

The question is then how to shape our societies and our lives to allow our social relationships to flourish. One answer is, of course, to focus on a healthy work–life balance. And many look at Denmark with envy when it comes to this. "We were not surprised to read last week that the Danes topped the UN's first World Happiness Report," Cathy Strongman wrote in *The Guardian*. She had moved from Finsbury Park in London to Copenhagen three years earlier, with her husband and their daughter.

Our quality of life has skyrocketed and our once staunch London loyalism has been replaced by an almost embarrassing enthusiasm for everything "Dansk." The greatest change has been the shift in work–life balance. Whereas previously we might snatch dinner once Duncan escaped from work at around nine, he now leaves his desk at five. Work later than 5.30, and the office is a morgue. Work at the weekend, and the Danes think you are mad. The idea is that families have time to play and eat together at the end of the day, every day. And it works. Duncan bathes and puts our 14-month-old daughter Liv to bed most nights. They are best buddies, as opposed to strangers who try to reacquaint at the weekend.

Cathy Strongman, The Guardian

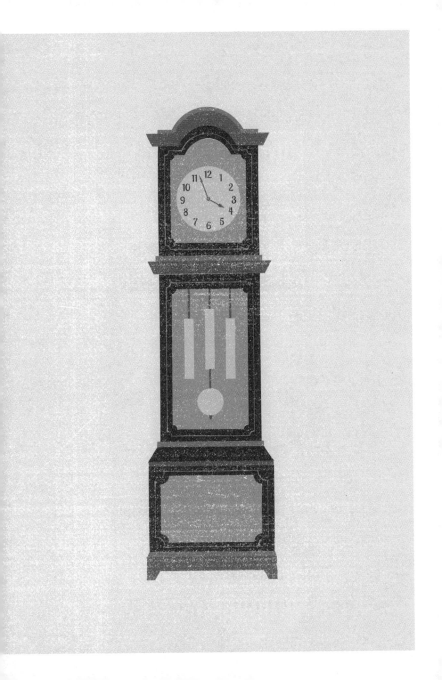

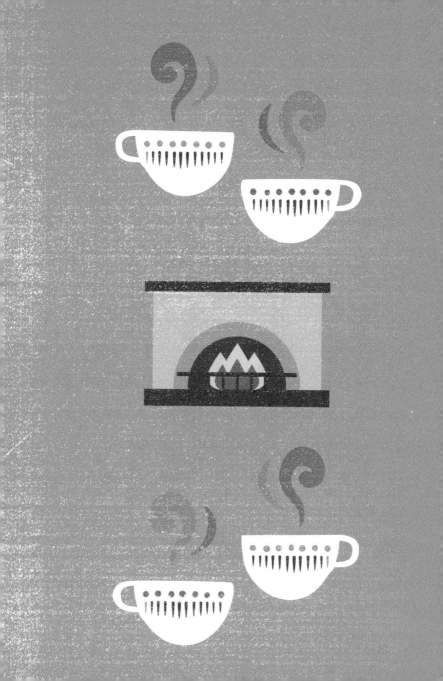

Some have described the Danish workplace as something like the opening credits of *The Flintstones*. Come five o'clock, everyone has left before you can say "Yabba dabba doo!" People with children usually leave at four; those without, at five. Everybody leaves, heading home to cook dinner. As a manager, I avoid scheduling meetings that would end after four if I have parents on my team, so they can pick up their kids at the usual time.

On average, 60 percent of Europeans socialize with friends, family, or colleagues a minimum of once a week. The corresponding average in Denmark is 78 percent. While you can hygge by yourself, hygge mostly happens in small groups of close friends or family.

Hygge is also a situation where there is a lot of relaxed thoughtfulness. Nobody takes center stage or dominates the conversation for long stretches of time. Equality is an important element in hygge—a trait that is deeply rooted in the Danish culture—and also manifests itself in the fact that everybody takes part in the chores of the *hyggelig* evening. It is more *hyggeligt* if we all help to prepare food, instead of having the host alone in the kitchen.

Time spent with others creates an atmosphere that is warm, relaxed, friendly, down-to-earth, close, comfortable, snug, and welcoming. In many ways, it is like a good hug, but without the physical contact. It is in this situation that you can be completely relaxed and yourself. The art of hygge is therefore also the art of expanding your comfort zone to include other people.

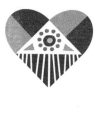

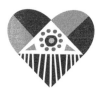

WHAT'S LOVE GOT TO DO WITH IT? OXYTOCIN

Someone puts a hand on your shoulder, gives you a kiss, or caresses your cheek and you instantly feel calm and happy. Our bodies work like that: it is a wonderful thing. Touch releases the hormone oxytocin, which makes us feel happy and reduces stress, fear, and pain.

But when do we experience the pleasure of having oxytocin flowing through our body? A widespread saying is that hugs make us happier, and that is true—oxytocin starts flowing in intimate situations, and helps us connect to each other. Therefore, it is also called "the cuddle hormone" or the "love hormone." Hygge is an intimate activity often connected with coziness and some company, which leads one to the conclusion that the body will make oxytocin flow during these events. Cuddling pets has the same effect as cuddling another person—we feel loved, warm, and safe, which are three key words in the concept of hygge. Oxytocin is released when we're physically close to another person's body, and can be described as a "social glue," since it keeps society together by means of cooperation, trust, and love. Maybe that is why Danes trust complete strangers to such a great extent; they hygge a lot, and *hyggelige* activities release oxytocin, which decreases hostility and increases social connection. Also, warmth and fullness release this hormone. Good food, candles, fireplaces, and blankets are constant companions to hygge. In a way, hygge is all about oxytocin. Could it be that simple? Perhaps it is not a coincidence that everything that has to do with hygge makes us feel happy, calm, and safe.

HAPPY TOGETHER

Being with other people is a key part of hygge, but as a happiness researcher, I can also testify that it might be the most important ingredient to happiness. There is broad agreement among happiness researchers and scientists that social relations are essential for people's happiness.

According to the World Happiness Report commissioned by the United Nations, "While basic living standards are essential for happiness, after the baseline has been met, happiness varies more with quality of human relationships than income."

The importance of our relationships has even led to attempts to evaluate them in monetary terms. "Putting a Price Tag on Friends, Relatives, and Neighbors: Using Surveys of Life Satisfaction to Value Social Relationships," a study undertaken in the United Kingdom in 2008, estimated that an increase in social involvements may produce an increase of life satisfaction equivalent to an extra $110,000 a year.

I see this link between our relationships and our happiness again and again, in global data and surveys, as well as Danish ones. One example is a city study we conducted a few years ago at the Happiness Research Institute, in the town of Dragør, just outside Copenhagen.

We were working with the city council to measure happiness and life satisfaction among the citizens. Together, we developed recommendations on how to improve quality of life in the city. As part of the exploration, we surveyed both how satisfied people were with their social relationships and how happy they were overall. Here we found—as we always do—a very strong correlation. The more satisfied people are with their social relationships, the happier they are in general. As I mentioned before, the relationship factor is usually the best predictor of whether people are happy or not. If I cannot ask people directly how happy they are, I ask them how satisfied they are with their social relationships, because that gives me the answer.

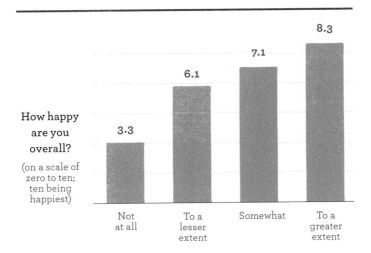

How happy are you overall?

(on a scale of zero to ten; ten being happiest)

3.3 — Not at all
6.1 — To a lesser extent
7.1 — Somewhat
8.3 — To a greater extent

How satisfied are you with your relationships?

An overall satisfaction with our relationships is one thing; the everyday joy of good company yet another. And here, Nobel Prize-winning psychologist Daniel Kahneman's Day Reconstruction Method may shed some light on the effect of hygge. The method prompts people to go through a normal day, rating how pleased or annoyed or depressed they feel during a range of activities.

In what has become a classic study from 2004, a group of scientists at Princeton, led by Dr. Kahneman, had 909 women in Texas participate in an experiment. The women would fill out a long diary and questionnaire detailing everything they had done the day before and rating it on a seven-point scale: what did they do and at what time, who were they with, and how did they feel during each activity? Perhaps unsurprisingly, the group of researchers found that commuting to work, doing housework, and facing a boss were among the least pleasant activities, while sex, socializing, eating and relaxing were the most enjoyable. Of course, socializing, eating, and relaxing are also main ingredients of hygge.

According to the "belongingness hypothesis", we have a basic need to feel connected with others, and close, caring bonds with other people play a major part in our motivation and behavior. Among the evidence for the belongingness hypothesis is the fact that people across the world are born with the ability and motivation to form close relationships, that people are reluctant to break bonds once they have been formed, and that married or cohabiting people live longer than single people (although this last is in part due to an enhanced immune system).

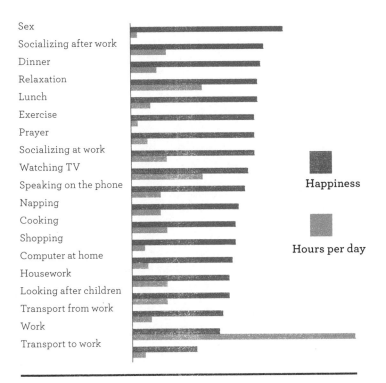

Sex
Socializing after work
Dinner
Relaxation
Lunch
Exercise
Prayer
Socializing at work
Watching TV
Speaking on the phone
Napping
Cooking
Shopping
Computer at home
Housework
Looking after children
Transport from work
Work
Transport to work

Happiness

Hours per day

Source: Kahneman et al., "A Survey Method for Characterizing Daily Life
Experience: The Day Reconstruction Method," *Science* 306 (December 3, 2004).

"Our relationships affect our happiness! Well, gosh, thank you, happiness research!" Yes, as scientists, we can find it quite frustrating to spend years looking into the question of why some people are happier than others and then find an answer that we all knew anyway. Nevertheless, now we have the numbers, the data, and the evidence to support the notion, and we can and should make use of them when we shape our policies, our societies, and our lives.

We are social creatures, and the importance of this is clearly seen when one compares the satisfaction people feel in relationships with their overall satisfaction with life. The most important social relationships are close relationships in which you experience things together with others, and experience being understood; where you share thoughts and feelings, and both give and receive support. In one word: hygge.

That may be why Danes prefer smaller circles of friends when they are looking for hygge. Of course, you can have a *hyggelig* time if there are more people, but Danes would rather a smaller group of people for a *hyggelig* time. Almost 60 percent of Danes say the best number of people for hygge is three to four.

How many does it take to hygge?

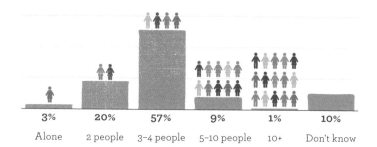

3%	20%	57%	9%	1%	10%
Alone	2 people	3–4 people	5–10 people	10+	Don't know

THE DARK SIDE
OF HYGGE

———

Hanging out with your close friends in a tightly knit social network, where you all go way back together and know each other well, definitely has its benefits.

But in recent years I have also come to realize that there is a severe drawback to a social landscape like this: it doesn't readily admit newcomers. Every person I've met who has moved to Denmark tells me the same thing. It is close to impossible to penetrate the social circles there. Or at least it requires years and years of hard work and persistence.

Admittedly, Danes are not good at inviting new people into their friendship circles. In part, this is due to the concept of hygge; it would be considered less *hyggeligt* if there were too many new people at an event. So getting into a social circle requires a lot of effort and a lot of loneliness on the way. The good thing is, in the words of my friend Jon, "Once you are in, you are in." Once you have broken through, you can trust you will have formed lifelong friendships.

HYGGE—SOCIALIZING FOR INTROVERTS

―――――

While I was researching this book, I gave a lecture to a group of American students who were spending a term in Copenhagen. I often use lectures as opportunities to gather input and inspiration for what I am currently researching, and this was no different, so I steered the discussion on toward relationship between well-being and hygge.

One student who had been quiet in the previous discussions raised her hand. "I am an introvert," she said. "And, to me, hygge is such a wonderful thing." Her point was that in the United States, she was used to taking part in social activities with a lot of people, a lot of fast networking, and much excitement. In short, she was in the realm of the extroverts. In Denmark, she found that the way social activities are organized suited her much more—and that hygge was the best thing that could happen for introverts. It was a way of being social without being draining for them. I thought that this was perhaps the most insightful thing I had heard in a long time and promised her I would steal her insight and put it in this book.

It is known that introverts derive their energy from within, while extroverts derive theirs from external stimulation. Introverts are often seen as loners, while extroverts are the ones to surround yourself with if you want to have a good time. Introversion is often wrongly linked with shyness, and although social events are not for everyone and might leave an introvert overstimulated and exhausted, social introverts do exist (just as calm extroverts do).

This may sound a bit clichéd, but introverts often prefer to devote their "social time" to loved ones whom they know very well, to have meaningful conversations or to sit down and read a book with something warm to drink. This happens to have a very high hygge factor—great, right? Introverts are social, but in a different way. There is not one single way of being social, but it might feel like there are right and wrong ways. Just because introverts are drained by too many external stimuli doesn't mean they don't want to hang out with other people. Hygge is a way of socializing that can suit introverts: they can have a relaxing and cozy night with a couple of friends without having to include a lot of people and a lot of activity. Introverts might want to stay at home instead of attending a big party with a lot of people they don't know, and hygge becomes an option, something in between socializing and relaxing. It makes these two worlds go hand in hand, which is great news for both introverts and extroverts, since it becomes something of a compromise. So, to all you introverts out there, do not feel embarrassed or boring for being a person who prefers things that are hygge. And to all extroverts: light some candles, put on some soothing music, and embrace your inner introvert, just for the night.

HYGGE TIP: HOW TO MAKE MEMORIES

It is common knowledge that the best part of memories is making them. Start a new tradition with your friends or family. It might be playing board games on the first Friday of every month, or celebrating the summer solstice by the water. In fact it can be whatever meaningful activity will knit the group more tightly together over the years.

CHAPTER FOUR

—

FOOD AND DRINK

YOU ARE WHAT YOU EAT

If hygge was a person, I think it would be Alice Waters. With a casual, rustic, and slow approach to life, she embodies many of the key elements of hygge—and she also seems to understand the value of good, hearty food in the company of good people.

New Nordic food has gotten a lot of attention in the last few years. The center of attention has been Noma, which opened in 2003 and has been rated the best restaurant in the world four times since 2010. While a dish consisting of live shrimp covered in ants may make the headlines, it is relatively far from everyday Danish cuisine. Traditional Danish lunch includes a budget version of *smørrebrød* (open-faced sandwiches) on rye bread with pickled herring or *leverpostej* (liver paste—a spreadable mixture of baked, chopped pig's liver and lard). I bet you think those ants are beginning to look appetizing. For dinner, *50 Shades of Meat and Potatoes* would be an apt title for a traditional Danish cookbook. Danes are meat lovers, and on average, every person consumes around 105 pounds of meat per year—with pork being the nation's favorite.

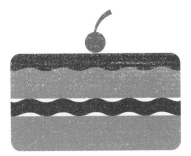

The high level of meat, confectionery and coffee consumption in Denmark is directly linked to hygge. Hygge is about being kind to yourself—giving yourself a treat, and giving yourself, and each other, a break from the demands of healthy living. Sweets are *hyggelige*. Cake is *hyggeligt*. Coffee or hot chocolate are *hyggeligt*, too. Carrot sticks, not so much. Something sinful is an integral component of the hygge ritual. But it should not be something fancy or extravagant. Foie gras is not *hyggeligt*. But a hearty stew is. Popcorn is. Especially if we all share the same bowl.

LET'S SIN TOGETHER

A couple of years ago, I visited a friend of mine and his family. His daughter was four at the time, and over dinner she turned to me and asked, "What is your job?"

"I try to find what makes people happy," I replied.

"That's easy." She shrugged. "Sweets." When it comes to happiness, I am not sure the answer is that simple, but she might have been onto something when it comes to hygge.

Danes are crazy about confectionery, and a majority of people associate it with hygge: gummy bears, licorice and *flødeboller* [fleu-the-ball-r], chocolate domes stuffed with cream. In fact, according to a report by Sugar Confectionery Europe, the annual consumption of confectionery in Denmark is 18 pounds per person, making Danes second only to the Finns as the people who eat more sweets than anyone in the world, twice the European average. Also, by 2018, Denmark is expected to overtake Finland as the world's most sweet-crazed country. And it is not just sweets Danes are crazy about. Cake, anyone?

Consumption of sweets

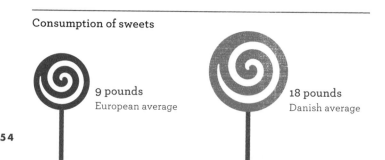

9 pounds
European average

18 pounds
Danish average

CAKE

Cake is most definitely hyggeligt, *and we Danes eat a lot of it. Cake is a common sight in our offices. Jon is one of my poker buddies, and he and I meet over a pint at his favorite bar in Copenhagen, Lord Nelson, to discuss hygge and our Danish cake obsession.*

"We do walks by the meeting rooms to scout and monitor left-over cake. We call it cake watch," he told me. "And this is just for internal meetings. If clients are coming, then there will be petits fours on top." Jon is right. Cakes and pastries make everything *hyggeligt*, both eating them and baking them. They also bring an atmosphere of casualness to any business meeting.

However, most cakes are eaten outside the office, at home or in cake shops. One of the most popular and traditional ones is La Glace, Denmark's oldest confectionery shop, established in 1870. Their selection of cakes, including cakes named after famous Danes like Hans Christian Andersen and Karen Blixen, looks like something out of a dream. Their most famous cake is perhaps "sport cake," which is essentially an ocean of whipped cream and so not exactly the breakfast of sports champions. The name derives from the fact that the cake was first produced for the premiere of a play called *Sports Man* in 1891. The old ideals, the interior, the cakes and pastries and the beautiful rooms in which one sits down to enjoy a sweet masterpiece scream hygge all over Copenhagen.

KAGEMAND

They say that your superheroes say a lot about you. Americans have Superman, Spiderman, and Batman. Danes have ... well ... Cakeman.

Okay, so he is not a superhero per se, but he is as popular as his American colleagues at birthday parties. Cakeman (*Kagemand* [Cai-man]) is a traditional element at Danish birthday parties for children. It looks like a large-scale gingerbread man, is made of a sweet dough with lots of sugar and butter, and is decorated with sweets, Danish flags, and candles. If only we could add bacon to the recipe, we would have all things essentially Danish in one place. Part of the tradition is that the birthday boy or girl cuts the throat of the Cakeman while the other kids scream.

> *"Happy birthday, darling. Now cut the throat of Cakeman." How is that for a hyggelig Nordic-noir birthday?*

PASTRIES

A pastry that is typically Danish is ... well ... a Danish. It is not every nationality that gets a butter-infused dough with gooey cream in the middle named after it.

Usually, it is the kind of nation that has lost every war they have participated in for centuries. However, in Denmark, Danish pastries are called *wienerbrød* (Vienna bread), as Danish pastry recipes were first developed by chefs who had been to Vienna in the middle of the nineteenth century. Some of the pastries have charming names such as "snails" or "the baker's bad eye," but names aside, they are delicious and good for hygge. Also, if you are looking to spread joy and cheer in a Danish office, just shout out the word *"Bon-kringle!" Kringle* is a classic Danish pastry and *bon* means receipt. The concept behind *bon-kringle* is that when you buy cake and pastry worth 1,000 kroner (around $140) at your local bakery, if you present the receipts, the baker will give you a free *kringle*. It's like a pastry loyalty card—but without the loyalty card.

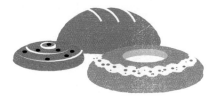

DIY

Getting your hands dirty by baking at home is a hyggelig *activity that you can do by yourself or with friends and family. Few things contribute more to the hygge factor than the smell of freshly baked goods.*

The result does not need to look like something out of a Disney movie—in fact, the more rustic, the more hygge it is. For some time now, sourdough has been a hit among a lot of Danes. The slowness of the process and the feeling of taking care of a living thing makes it all the more *hyggeligt*. Some Danes talk about their dough as if it were their baby, which they feed and care for. Sourdough is basically a gastronomic alternative to The Sims.

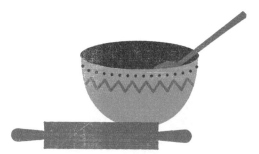

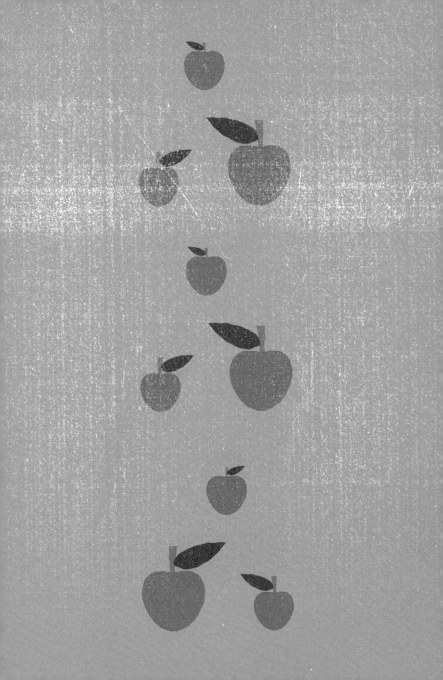

HOT DRINKS

My team of researchers ran a survey among Danes to find out what people associate hygge with. I had put my money on candles, but I was wrong. Candles came second, while hot drinks took first place.

Hot drinks are what 86 percent of Danes associate with hygge. It might be tea, hot chocolate, or mulled wine, but the Danes' favorite hot drink is coffee.

If you love Danish TV dramas like *Borgen* or *The Killing*, you will be familiar with the Danes' love of coffee. Hardly a scene goes by without someone ordering a coffee, brewing coffee, or one person looking at another while asking, "Coffee?" Danes are the world's fourth biggest coffee drinkers and consume around 33 percent more per capita than Americans.

> *"Live life today like there is no coffee tomorrow."*

The link between coffee and hygge is evident in the Danish language. *Kaffehygge*, another compound word, this one consisting of *coffee* and *hygge*, is everywhere. "Come to *kaffehygge*," *kaffehygge* and cake, workout and *kaffehygge*, yarn and *kaffehygge*. *Kaffehygge* is everywhere. There is even a website dedicated to *kaffehygge* that states, "Live life today like there is no coffee tomorrow."

So while you can hygge without coffee, having some definitely helps. There is something comforting about having a warm cup of coffee in your hands. It is definitely conducive to hygge.

ADDICTED TO HYGGE?

You can't buy happiness, but you can buy cake, and that is almost the same thing—at least, that might be our brain's opinion. Imagine opening the door to a coffee shop. Tempting aromas from all the sweet things on the counter hit you as you step inside, and when you see all the pastries and cakes you feel happy. You choose your favorite cake, and when you take the first bite, a feeling of euphoria spreads through your body. Oh yes, that is good. But have you thought about *why* you feel so happy when eating sugary food?

What do Danes associate with hygge?

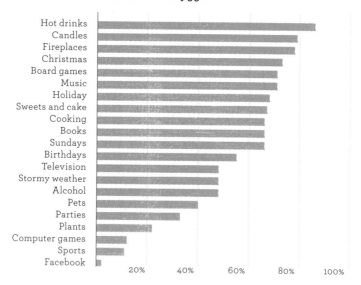

In the basal forebrain there is something called the nucleus accumbens. It is a part of the brain's reward system and has a significant role when it comes to motivation, pleasure, and reinforcement. Like all other vertebrates, we have this system because it is important that we feel pleasure when doing things like eating food and having sex, since these things are vital for our species' survival.

When you are doing something that is considered rewarding, a chemical substance is released in the brain, and the signal substance dopamine is activated. Close to the nucleus accumbens, there is an area called the ventral tegmental area, and dopamine is released from there in reward situations. It is when dopamine is transferred from nerve fibers to receptors in different parts of the brain that we experience pleasure. Memories of a pleasurable event are stored in the cerebral cortex so we won't forget them. It may sound strange, but in a way, you could say the brain creates addictions for our survival.

When we are born, the first thing we taste is sweet breast milk. Liking sweet food is beneficial for our survival, and that is why we experience feelings of joy when eating cakes and other sugary things, and why we find it hard to stop. Our body has taught us to continue doing things that are rewarded. It's the same thing that calls when it comes to fat and salt.

In short, we associate a certain kind of food with the feeling of pleasure, which makes us want more. Hygge is something that is supposed to be and feel good for you, and that means if you want to eat cake, have some cake. But at the same time, we must know when to stop. It is not very *hyggeligt* to have a stomachache.

SLOW FOOD'S CHUBBY COUSIN

So confectionery, cakes, and pastries are hyggelige. *But there is more to hygge food than increasing your body mass. Hygge may be comfort food. But hygge food is also very much slow food.*

How *hyggelig* a food is also lies in its preparation. The rule of thumb is: the longer a dish takes to cook, the more *hyggelig* it is.

Preparing hygge food is about enjoying the slow process of it, about appreciating the time you spend and the joy of preparing something of value. It is about your relationship with the meal. That is why homemade jams are more *hyggelige* than bought ones. Every bite will take you back to that summer day when you picked the fruit and the entire house smelled of strawberries.

Especially in the wintertime, I enjoy spending the best part of a weekend afternoon cooking something that requires hours baking in the oven or simmering on the stove. The process can even be extended by visiting a great farmers' market, carefully selecting the vegetables in season or having a chat with the butcher about which meat he would recommend for a slow-cooked stew. Having a pot simmering on the stove while you are reading a book in your *hyggekrog* is not only the sound of hygge but the essence of hygge. The only reason to get up is to add a bit more red wine to the stew.

It is important to stress that the process need not revolve around the simmering of some meaty old Nordic cuisine. It is about the process, not the end product. Last summer, I tried to make limoncello. Part of the process is that you leave the peel of several lemons soaking in alcohol for over a week, for the alcohol to absorb the flavor and the color of the peel. Every day after work I would come home, open the fridge, and take a good sniff to see how my concoction was progressing. The end result was so-so, but the enjoyment from monitoring the progress of the bottle in the fridge was hygge all the way.

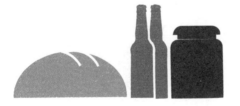

HYGGE RECIPES

—

Five recipes that will definitely get the hygge going.

SKIBBERLABSKOVS

BRAISED PORK CHEEKS IN DARK BEER WITH POTATO-CELERIAC MASH

BOLLER I KARRY

GLØGG

SNOBRØD

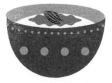

SKIBBERLABSKOVS
(SKIP-ER-LAP-SCOWS)

SKIPPER STEW

This dish is a hearty down-to-earth stew, originally made
on ships (hence the name), and is great for a brisk autumn day.
Instead of brisket, you can use leftover meat, making it even
more down-to-earth and *hyggelig*.

Serves 4–6. Cooking time 1 hour and 15 minutes.

1½ pounds brisket

3 onions

7 tablespoons butter

3–4 bay leaves

10–12 black peppercorns

4 cups chicken stock

3½ pounds potatoes

Salt and pepper

A handful of chives

4–6 pickled beets

Rye bread

1. Cut the brisket into bite-size cubes.

2. Peel and chop the onions.

3. Melt the butter in a thick-bottomed pot or Dutch oven and sauté the onions until they are translucent (they should not brown).

4. Add the meat, bay leaves, and peppercorns, then pour the boiling chicken stock into the pot. It should just cover the meat and onions.

5. Cover and leave to simmer for about forty-five minutes. Peel the potatoes and cut them into bite-size pieces.

6. Put half of the potatoes on top of the meat and put the lid back on.

7. After fifteen minutes, stir the contents of the pot and add the rest of the potatoes—and a bit of extra chicken stock if needed. Simmer for another fifteen to twenty minutes on low heat, remembering to stir frequently so the stew doesn't burn on the bottom. The aim is for the meat to be sitting in a potato mash but for there still to be whole pieces of tender potato.

8. Season with salt and pepper, and serve hot with a pat of butter, a generous amount of chives, one pickled beet per person, and rye bread.

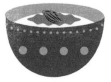

BRAISED PORK CHEEKS IN DARK BEER WITH POTATO-CELERIAC MASH

This is one of my favorite winter dishes. It needs to simmer for a long time on the stove to increase the hygge factor, and to allow you to spend time with a glass of wine and your favorite book in the meantime.

Serves 4. Cooking time 1 hour and 45 minutes–2 hours.

For the braised pork cheeks:

10–12 pork cheeks

Salt and pepper

1 tablespoon butter

⅛ celeriac, peeled and roughly chopped

1 carrot, peeled and roughly chopped

1 onion, peeled and roughly chopped

1 tomato, quartered

1 pint of dark beer or ale

For the potato-celeriac mash:

1¾ pounds potatoes

¼ celeriac, peeled

scant 1 cup milk

2 tablespoons butter

Handful chopped parsley and bread for serving

Braised pork cheeks:

1. Dry the pork cheeks with a paper towel and season with the salt and pepper.

2. Let the butter turn golden in a saucepan over medium to high heat. Add the meat and brown it on all sides, roughly three to four minutes in total.

3. Add the celeriac, carrot, and onion and let them brown before adding the tomato.

4. Pour in the beer. Add water if necessary to cover the meat and vegetables.

5. Turn the heat down low and simmer for about an hour and a half, until the meat is tender.

6. Remove the meat but continue boiling to reduce the sauce, then put it through a sieve and season.

Potato-celeriac mash:

1. Cut the potatoes and celeriac into bite-size pieces.

2. Boil the potatoes and celeriac until tender, then drain and mash the vegetables.

3. Warm the milk in the pan, and add it and the butter to the mash. Season.

4. Serve the braised pork cheeks on a bed of mash. You may add a sprinkle of parsley and some bread* to mop up the sauce.

---

* Use sourdough for maximum hygge, but any bread that works as a good sauce mop will do.

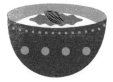

BOLLER I KARRY
[BALL-R E CARI]

DANISH MEATBALLS IN CURRY

This traditional Danish recipe is very popular among
Danes of all ages. This was my mother's favorite dish and, even
though she died almost twenty years ago, I still make it every year
on her birthday. What better way of remembering the ones we have
lost than by cooking their favorite meal? It can turn a sad occasion
into a *hyggelig* evening. Do not be concerned if you are not
a fan of spicy food. This is a very mildly spiced dish,
and many Danish kids are big fans.

**Serves 4. Cooking time 1 hour and 35 minutes
(including 1 hour for the mix to rest).**

1 cup breadcrumbs, or
2 tablespoons flour

1 egg

2 onions, peeled and finely
chopped

3 garlic cloves

Salt and pepper

4 ½ pounds ground pork

4 cups beef stock

For the curry sauce:

2 tablespoons butter

2 heaping tablespoons of mild yellow curry powder

1 large onion, peeled and chopped

1 large leek, peeled and finely chopped

5 tablespoons flour

½ cup heavy cream

Handful chopped fresh parsley

---

1. Place the bread crumbs or flour with the egg, onions, garlic, salt, and pepper in a big bowl and mix it well. Add the pork, mix it again, and leave in the fridge for one hour.

2. Take the mixture out of the fridge and use a spoon to form little balls. Add water to a cooking pot and bring it to a boil over high heat. Add the beef stock and the meatballs into the boiling water and let them simmer for five to ten minutes. Remove the meatballs from the water, but retain some of the liquid for later use.

3. Melt the butter in a pot, add the curry powder, and let it brown for a couple of minutes.

4. Add the chopped onion and leek and let them brown for a couple of minutes. Add flour and mix well. Then add some of the cooking liquid, little by little, stirring until the sauce thickens. Add the cream and the meatballs and simmer for about twelve minutes.

5. Garnish with parsley and serve with rice.

GLØGG
(GLOEG)

MULLED WINE

No December is complete without the traditional *gløgg*.
Danes will meet at bars or invite friends and family over to wish
each other a Merry Christmas over this warm, spicy wine.

**Serves 6–10. Cooking time 20 minutes
(plus soaking time for raisins)**

For the *gløgg* essence:

4 handfuls of raisins

10 ounces port

1 bottle of heavy red wine, such
as Beaujolais or Côtes du Rhone*

1 cup brown sugar (preferably

a brown sugar that consists of
sugar crystals and cane syrup—
but normal brown sugar will do)

20g cinnamon sticks
(8 to 10 sticks)

20g allspice (whole)

20g cloves (whole)

10g cardamom (whole)

---

* Don't go for the cheapest ones, but
there is no need to spend all your savings
for mulled wine either.

For the gløgg:

2 bottles of heavy red wine, such as Beaujolais or Côtes du Rhone

¾ cup brown rum

¾ cup akvavit (or vodka)

Peel of 1 orange

¾ cup freshly squeezed orange juice

1 cup chopped almonds

---

1. Soak the raisins in the port, preferably for 24 hours.

2. Start by making the *gløgg* essence. Pour the bottle of red wine into a pot, add the sugar and cinnamon, allspice, cloves, and cardamom, and heat to just below boiling point. Turn off the heat and allow to cool, then strain out the aromatics.

3. Add the additional bottles of red wine, spirits, orange peel and juice to the *gløgg* essence. Again, heat to just below boiling point, and then add the raisins, port and the almonds. Serve warm.

SNOBRØD
(SNO-BROEÐ)*

TWISTBREAD

This dish is not likely to be featured at Noma any time soon.
It is not the fanciest bread you'll ever have, but the process of
making it gets top marks for hygge and kids love it.

Makes 6 pieces.

**Cooking time 1 hour and 15 minutes
(including 1 hour for the dough to rest).**

2 tablespoons butter

1 cup milk

6½ teaspoons yeast

2 teaspoons sugar

¾ teaspoon salt

3⅛ cup flour

---

* This soft ð is one of the most difficult Danish sounds. The closest it comes to
English is th, but with your tongue extended a little further.

1. Melt the butter in a saucepan and add the milk. Heat until lukewarm. Add the yeast and dissolve.

2. Pour the mix into a large bowl and add the other ingredients to make a dough, but save a little bit of the flour. Knead the dough well and put it back into the bowl. Cover and leave it to rise for about an hour in a warm place.

3. Put the dough on a flour-covered surface and knead well again. You may add the rest of the flour at this point. Divide the dough into six pieces and roll each piece into a strip about 16 inches long, then wind around a thickish stick.

4. Bake the bread over the embers of a fire, but be careful not to have the bread too close to the heat. The bread will be baked sufficiently when it gives a hollow sound when you knock on it, or when it easily slips off the stick. Baking time depends on the fire and your patience, but usually around ten minutes.

HYGGE TIP: CREATE A COOKING CLUB

A few years ago, I wanted to create some kind of system that would mean I would get to see some of my good friends on a regular basis, so we formed a cooking club. This was in part prompted by my work, as the importance of our relationships always emerges as a key indicator of why some people are happier than others. Furthermore, I wanted to organize the cooking club in a way that maximized the hygge. So instead of taking turns being the host and cooking for the five or six other people, we always cook together. That is where the hygge is. The rules are simple. Each time there is a theme, or a key ingredient—for example, duck or sausages—each person brings ingredients to make a small dish to fit the theme. It creates a very relaxed, informal, egalitarian setting, where no one person has to cater for the guests—or live up to the standards of the last fancy dinner party.

One of the most *hyggelig* evenings we have had in the cooking club was the time we tried to make sausages. We spent three or four hours mincing the meat, stuffing the casings, boiling and frying the sausages. Feeling proud of ourselves, we were looking at mountains of sausages when we were finally able to sit down, around ten o'clock in the evening, hungry as Vikings. The result: disastrous. The first taste sensation I got was mold. Not exactly what you are looking for in a sausage. We might have gone to bed slightly hungry that night—but the evening had been very *hyggelig*.

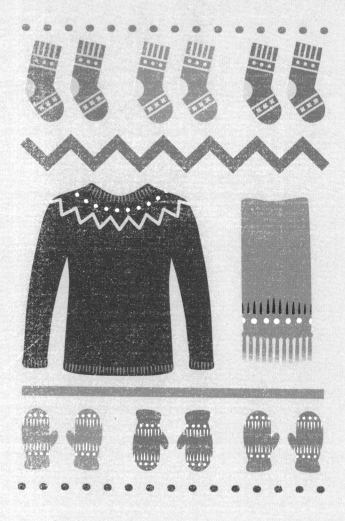

CHAPTER FIVE

—

CLOTHING

CASUAL IS KEY

When it comes to Denmark, casual is key. Danes in general enjoy a casual tone, a casual atmosphere, and a casual dress code.

You will not find many three-piece suits on the streets of Copenhagen, and if you are part of the pinstriped business brigade, you are bound to find the Danish way of dressing almost sloppy. However, you may in time discover that there is a Danish art to master being stylish and casual at the same time. For the casual yet stylish look, many people—including me—go with the combo of a T-shirt or sweater on the inside and then a blazer on the outside. I prefer the ones with leather patches on the elbows for the hygge and for the professor look. In fact, I may overuse the patches a little bit, as my friends joke that if they need to look for me when I am standing with my back to them in a crowded bar, they just look out for the patches.

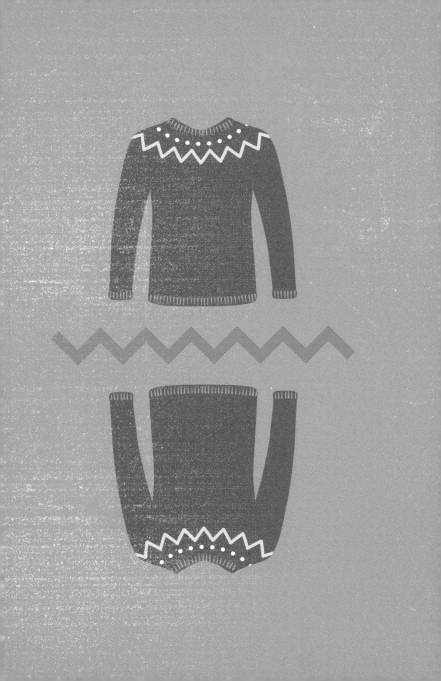

HOW TO DRESS LIKE
A DANE

Danish fashion is sleek, minimalistic, elegant, but not highly strung. In many ways, it is a sweet spot between hygge and minimalistic functional design.

SCARVES

A scarf is a must. This goes for men as well as women. While it is predominantly for the winter, people suffering from scarves withdrawal symptoms have been observed wearing scarves midsummer. The golden rule is: the bigger the better. So pile that stylish, thickly wrapped scarf on, just one step short of risking neck injuries. The Danes love scarves so much that some Brits have been referring to the Danish TV drama *Borgen* as "Scarf Watch."

BLACK

Once you get out of Copenhagen airport, you may think you have walked onto the set of a ninja movie. In Denmark, everyone wears black. You want to aim for a look that would be fitting for Karl Lagerfeld's funeral: stylish but monochrome. In the summertime, you are allowed to go for a wider range of colors, even something crazily flamboyant like gray.

TOP BULKY

A combination of hand-knitted wool sweaters, jumpers, cardigans, and pullovers on top, and black leggings for girls and skinny jeans for boys will give you the balance between hygge and fashion. Sweaters can be bulky but never sloppy—and don't forget the scarf.

LAYERS

The key to surviving four seasons in one day is layers. You should always bring another cardigan. You can't hygge when you are cold.

WOOLEN SOCKS

Ally yourself with a nice pair of woolen socks as a hygge insurance.

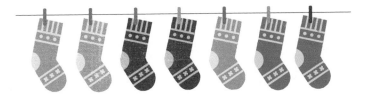

CASUAL HAIR

The Danish hairstyle is casual to the point of being borderline lazy. Wake up and go. Girls can put their hair in a bun, the higher the better.

THE SARAH LUND SWEATER

Perhaps the most iconic sweater is the one made famous by Sarah Lund in the Danish TV drama *The Killing. The Guardian* even featured an article entitled "*The Killing*: Sarah Lund's jumper explained." The sweater became so popular that the company producing it in the Faroe Islands couldn't keep up with demand.

It was the actress Sofie Gråbøl who chose the sweater. "I saw that sweater and thought, that's it! Lund is so sure of herself. She doesn't have to wear a suit. She's at peace with herself." The sweater is also a reminder of her childhood in the seventies and her hippie parents, who wore similar sweaters. "That sweater was a sign of believing in togetherness."

HYGGE TIP: HOW TO BUY

Link purchases with good experiences. I had saved money for a new favorite chair but waited until I had published my first book to get it. That way, the chair reminds me of something that was an important accomplishment for me. We can apply the same thing to that special sweater or that pair of nice woolen socks. Save for them—but wait until you have that really *hyggelig* experience: you want to be reminded of it when you pull them on.

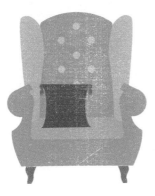

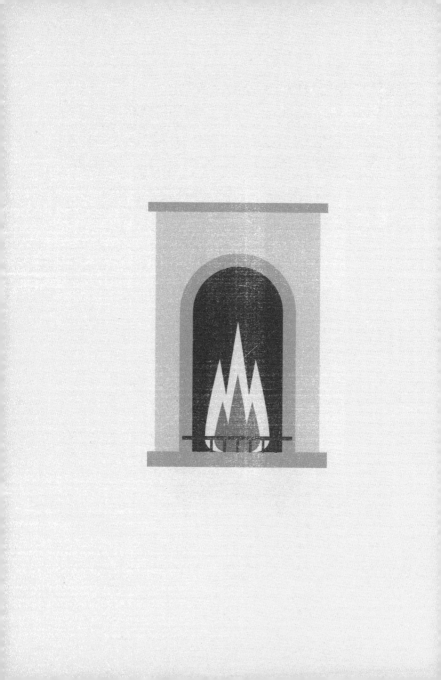

CHAPTER SIX

HOME

HYGGE HEADQUARTERS

Danish TV dramas such as Borgen, The Killing, *and* The Bridge *are, by people abroad, sometimes referred to as "furniture porn." Most scenes are shot in beautifully decorated houses and flats furnished with Danish design classics.*

And yes, Danes do love design, and walking into many Danish homes can be like walking into the pages of an interior design magazine.

The reason for the Danish obsession with interior design is that our homes are the hygge headquarters. Home is central to social life in Denmark. Whereas other countries have a culture of social life predominantly taking place in bars, restaurants, and cafés, Danes prefer *hjemmehygge* (home hygge)—among other reasons, to avoid the high prices charged in restaurants. Seven out of ten Danes say they experience most hygge at home.

Where do you experience the most hygge?

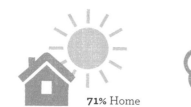
71% Home

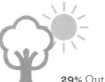
29% Out

Danes therefore tend to put a lot of effort and money into making their homes *hyggelige*. They enjoy the most living space per capita in all of Europe.

Square meters per resident

51	**44**	**44**	**41**	**40**	**38**
Denmark	Sweden	UK	Netherlands	Germany	France

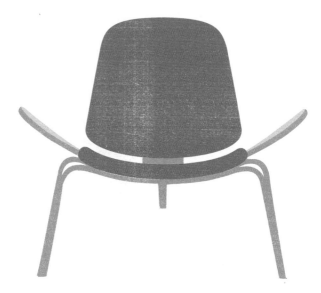

One December while I was a student, I spent all my spare time selling Christmas trees. It was a cold winter, but working with the trees kept me warm. I spent the entire salary I earned that month from carrying, sawing, hammering, chopping, and selling trees on a chair: the Shell Chair, a beauty designed in 1963 by Hans J. Wegner. Mine was walnut with dark brown leather. Two years later, my apartment was broken into. They stole the chair. Needless to say, I was angry that my beautiful chair had been stolen. But at least the burglars had good taste.

Perhaps the Danish obsession with design is best exemplified by what is now known as the Kähler Vase Scandal, or simply Vasegate. The Kähler vase was an anniversary piece that was sold in a limited edition on August 25, 2014. More than 16,000 Danes tried to buy it online that day—most in vain, as the vase quickly sold out. The website crashed and people queued in long lines outside the stores that were stocking the vase. The company that produced the vase was hit by a public backlash over the limited supply. Was this a little too much hysteria over an eight-inch-high vase with copper stripes, even though it would complement most Danish homes nicely? Perhaps, but Danes have relatively short working weeks, and get free health care and a university education on top of five weeks of paid holiday per year. Not getting that vase was the worst thing that had happened to them in years.

HYGGE WISHLIST:

TEN THINGS THAT WILL MAKE YOUR HOME MORE HYGELLIG

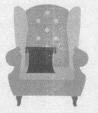

1. A HYGGEKROG.

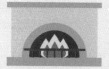

2. A FIREPLACE

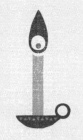

3. CANDLES

4. THINGS MADE OUT OF WOOD

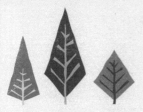

5. NATURE

6. BOOKS

7. CERAMICS

**8. THINK
TACTILE**

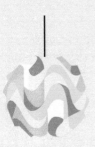

9. VINTAGE

**10. BLANKETS
AND CUSHIONS**

1. A HYGGEKROG

The one thing that every home needs is a *hyggekrog*, which roughly translates as "a nook." It is the place in the room where you love to snuggle up in a blanket, with a book and a cup of tea. Mine is by the kitchen window. I've put some cushions, a blanket, and a reindeer hide there, and I also sit there to work in the evenings. In fact, many of these pages were written there.

Danes love their comfy space. Everyone wants one, and *hyggekroge* are common in Copenhagen and throughout the country. Walking on the streets of the city, you will notice that many of the buildings have a bay window. On the inside, these are almost certainly filled with cushions and blankets, providing the people who live there with a cozy place to sit and relax after a long day.

Your *hyggekrog* does not need to be by the window, however, even though that is really *hyggeligt*. It could be a part of a room. Just add some cushions or something else that feels nice to sit on, have soft lighting, maybe a blanket, and you will have your own *hyggekrog*, where you can enjoy a good book and something to drink. To furnish *hyggeligt* is a big deal in Denmark. Some real estate agents even use a *hyggekrog* as a way to sell houses.

Our love of small spaces may, if we look back in time, go back to when we lived in caves and it was important to pay attention to your environment in order to protect yourself and your group against dangerous animals and other threats. Living in small spaces was preferable, since the warmth generated by the inhabitants' bodies did not disappear as fast as it would in a larger one; in addition, small spaces were great places to hide from predators. Today, one of the reasons we like to sit in a *hyggekrog* could be that it makes us feel safe; overlooking another room or the street gives us the advantage of spotting *any* potential threat. We feel relaxed when we're in a *hyggekrog*. We feel that we have control over our situation and do not feel exposed to the unpredictable.

2. A FIREPLACE

I was a fortunate child. My childhood home had an open fireplace *and* a wood-burning stove. As a kid, my favorite chore was to stack the firewood and light the fire. I am sure I am not the only one. According to the Danish Ministry for the Environment, there are around 750,000 fireplaces and wood-fired stoves in Denmark. With a little over 2.5 million homes in the country, that means that three out of ten homes in Denmark have a hygge advantage. In comparison, around a million homes in the United Kingdom have installed a wood stove, but with a total of 28 million British homes, that's only around one in twenty-eight.

In this regard, the US is well-positioned for hygge today. According to the National Association of Home Builders, 60 percent of new homes have at least one fireplace, compared with a third of homes built forty years ago. It is also one of the favorite amenities for potential buyers.

So what's the reason for the Danish obsession with burning logs? You've probably already guessed the answer to this one, but surely it can't only be about hygge? Well, according to a study conducted by the University of Aarhus, that is true: Danes have wood-burning stoves because they are considered a cheap heating option, but this is only the *second* biggest reason for having one. Once again, it's mostly about hygge. Sixty-six percent of all respondents in the study specifically addressed hygge as the most important reason for having a wood-burning *stove*. And if you ask Danes, 70 percent will agree that fireplaces are *hyggelig*. One respondent to the survey even called fireplaces the most *hyggelig* piece of applied art ever made.

It is fair to say that a fireplace may just be the ultimate headquarters of hygge. It's somewhere we sit by ourselves to rest while experiencing ultimate feelings of coziness and warmth, and it's somewhere we spend time with our dear ones to intensify our feeling of togetherness.

Homes with a fireplace or a stove

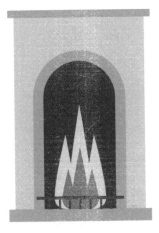
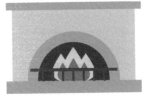

30%
Denmark

3.5%
UK

3. CANDLES

No candles, no hygge. If this is a surprise to you, you need to revisit Chapter 1.

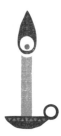

4. THINGS MADE OUT OF WOOD

Maybe we hanker after our roots, but there is just something about wooden things. The smell of burning wood from a fireplace, or even a match, the smooth feeling of a wooden bureau, the soft creak of a wooden floor as you trip across it to have a seat in the wooden chair by the window. Wooden children's toys have become popular again, after years of plastic toys. Kay Bojesen's wooden monkey is an excellent example of this. Wood makes us feel closer to nature; it is simple and natural, just like the concept of hygge.

5. NATURE

Wood is not enough. Danes feel the need to bring the entire forest inside. Any piece of nature you might find is likely to get the hygge greenlight. Leaves, nuts, twigs, animal skins. . . Basically, you want to think: How would a Viking squirrel furnish a living room? Be sure to smother those benches, chairs, and windowsills in sheepskin to give them an extra layer of hygge. You may alternate between sheep and reindeer, while keeping cowhides for the floor. With the Danes' love of candles and wooden and other flammable things, it is no surprise that Copenhagen has been burned to the ground on several occasions. Make sure fire precautions are taken.

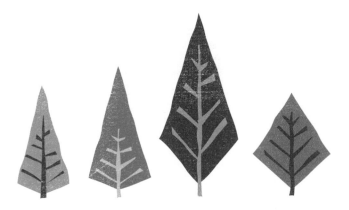

6. BOOKS

Who does not like a shelf filled with thick books? Taking a break with a good book is a cornerstone in the concept of hygge. The genre does not matter—romance, sci-fi, cookbooks, or even horror stories are welcome on the shelves. All books are *hyggelig*, but classics written by authors such as Jane Austen, Charlotte Brontë, Leo Tolstoy, and Charles Dickens have a special place on the bookshelf. At the right age, your kids may also love to cuddle up with you in the *hyggekrog* and have you read to them. Probably not Tolstoy, though.

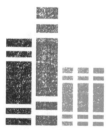

7. CERAMICS

A nice teapot, a vase on the dining table, that favorite mug you always want to drink out of—they are all *hyggelige*. Two of the most iconic Danish ceramics are Kähler, which goes back more than 175 years and made a big impression at the Universal Exposition in Paris in 1889—the year the Eiffel Tower was inaugurated—and of course Royal Copenhagen, founded in 1775 under the protection of Queen Juliane Marie, which has had a revival in popularity in recent years with the Blue Fluted Mega range.

8. THINK TACTILE

As you may have discovered by now, a *hyggelig* interior is not just about how things *look*, it is just as much about how things *feel*. Letting your fingers run across a wooden table, over a warm ceramic cup, or through the hairs of the skin of a reindeer is a distinctly different feeling from being in contact with something made from steel, glass, or plastic. Think about the way objects feel to your touch and add a variety of textures to your home.

9. VINTAGE

Vintage is a big deal in Danish homes, and you can find pretty much anything in a vintage or antiques shop. Often, the challenge is to find diamonds among a lot of coal. An old lamp, table, or chair is considered really *hyggeligt*. One can find everything one needs to create a lovely home in a vintage store, and the fact that all the things there have a history makes them even more interesting and *hyggelig*.

With many of these items, narratives and nostalgia come into play. Objects are more than their physical properties; they hold an emotional value and a story. I think my favorite pieces of furniture in my apartment are two footstools. My uncle and I made them together. I am sure I could find something similar in the shops around Copenhagen, but nothing that would mean the same to me. When I look at them, I remember that afternoon ten years ago when we carved them out of a branch of a hundred-year-old walnut tree. That is hygge. They allow you to sit comfortably with your legs up, plus they're made of wood and hold nostalgic value. They are, essentially, the Kinder egg of hygge.

10. BLANKETS AND CUSHIONS

Blankets and cushions are must-haves in any hygge household, especially during the cold months of winter. To snuggle up with a blanket is very *hyggeligt*, and sometimes one does it even though one is not feeling cold, simply because it is cozy. Blankets can be made out of fabrics such as wool or fleece, which are warmer, or cotton for a lighter feeling.

Large or small, cushions are also hygge essentials. What is better than leaning your head against a nice cushion while reading your favorite book?

At this point, you are welcome to go Freudian on the Danes and point out that hygge seems to be about comfort food and security blankets. And perhaps you are right. Hygge is about giving your responsible, stressed-out achiever adult a break. Relax. Just for a little while. It is about experiencing happiness in simple pleasures and knowing that everything is going to be okay.

HYGGE EMERGENCY KIT

You may also consider building a hygge emergency kit, stored up for those evenings when you are low on energy, have no plans, don't feel like going out, and are in the mood for some quality time alone.

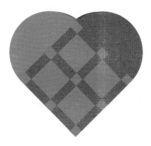

Have a box, cupboard or suitcase filled with hygge essentials. The list below might give you inspiration as to what you put in it, but of course it is completely up to you to decide and discover what you need for a fast track to hygge.

1. CANDLES

2. SOME GOOD-QUALITY CHOCOLATE

Why not visit the closest chocolatier and bring home a little box of high-quality chocolate? It doesn't have to be expensive, just a little treat to savor every now and then. If you are like me, make a contract with yourself that you can have one piece per day or per week;—otherwise it tends to disappear rather quickly. Having it as a weekly or daily ritual will give you a little pleasure to look forward to each day.

3. YOUR FAVORITE TEA

(Mine is currently rooibos).

4. YOUR FAVORITE BOOK

What book makes you forget the world and disappear in between the pages? Find out and put it in the emergency kit for those hygge evenings. If you have a job like mine, where you need to read a lot of stuff and quickly absorb the key points, you may tend to rush through the pages when you finally pick up fiction. We are tempted to turn immediately to the last page of the John le Carré spy novel: "Ah, what do you know? He was a double agent all along." Remember: this is a different kind of reading. Read slowly and see the story play out. My go-to book is *A Farewell to Arms by* Ernest Hemingway.

5. YOUR FAVORITE FILM OR TV SERIES

Mine is *Matador* (*Monopoly*), a Danish drama shot almost forty years ago, portraying life in a small town in Denmark from the Great Depression and through the Nazi occupation of Denmark. The series has become part of the modern self-understanding of Danes, and most Danish people will know at least a few of the lines.

6. JAM

There is something *hyggeligt* about jam, especially if you or someone you know has made it. So spend the summer conserving the fruit. Your hygge kit will thank you for it.

7. A GOOD PAIR OF WOOLEN SOCKS

8. A SELECTION OF YOUR FAVORITE LETTERS

The spoken word ceases to exist the moment it is born, but with the written language we are able to hear words from centuries ago or the words of loved ones far away. Rereading old letters is a *hyggelig* way of relaxing, remembering and reconnecting.

There is something more *hyggeligt* about a letter on paper than a letter on a screen. If you grew up in the last century, as I did, you'll have those handwritten letters safely stored away, but letters written in the Internet age may be printed and stored as well.

9. A WARM SWEATER

10. A NOTEBOOK

Keep a nice notebook in your hygge emergency kit. We may call this your hygge journal. The first exercise is to note down some of the most *hyggelige* moments you have experienced in the past month or year. This will allow you to enjoy them again and make you mindful of which experiences you enjoyed. For the second exercise, think of what kind of *hyggelige* experiences you would like to have in the future. A bucket list of hygge, if you will.

11. A NICE BLANKET

12. PAPER AND A PEN

It was nice and *hyggeligt* to read those old letters, wasn't it? Why not return the favor? Take the time to write a handwritten letter. Think of someone who you are grateful to have in your life and write to them to tell them why.

13. MUSIC

Vinyl would be considered more *hyggelig* than digital, but services like iTunes and Spotify allow you to create a hygge playlist that's up and running. I would go for something slow. Lately, I've been listening a lot to Gregory Alan Isakov and Charles Bradley, but you may want to go with the Danish artist Agnes Obel.

14. A PHOTO ALBUM

You know all those photos you uploaded on Facebook? Why not select a hundred of your favorite pictures and have them printed? An album of printed photos is much more *hyggelig* to browse through on a stormy night with a mug of tea.

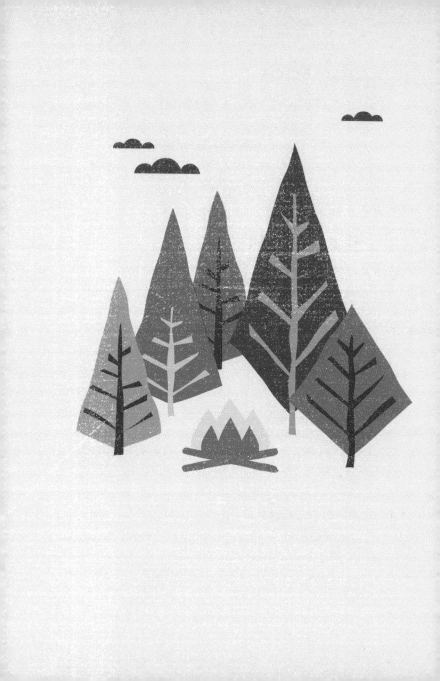

CHAPTER SEVEN

HYGGE OUTSIDE THE HOME

🌳🌳🌳🌳🌳🌳🌳🌳

THE GREAT OUTDOORS

———

While homes may be central for hygge, it is definitely possible to have hygge outside the home. In fact, cabins, boats, and the great outdoors are excellent places to experience hygge. Anywhere, at any time, can be hygge, but I've noticed that hygge moments are created by one or many of these key hygge drivers.

THE HYGGE DRIVERS

As a scientist, my work often involves looking for patterns in the evidence. So, if we look at cases of hyggelige, _we also find some common denominators for these moments of hygge. (I think we have already covered food and candles extensively enough, so we will leave these out for now.)_

COMPANY

You can hygge by yourself. Snuggling up under a blanket with your favorite TV show on a rainy Sunday afternoon is _hyggeligt_; having a glass of red wine watching a thunderstorm is _hyggeligt_ too, or simply just sitting by the window watching the world go by.

But the most _hyggelige_ moments seem to happen in the company of other people. A few years ago, my dad and his two brothers turned two hundred years combined, so they rented a big summer cabin on the west coast of Denmark and invited the whole family. The cabin was surrounded by sand dunes and was set in a rough, rugged landscape where the wind always blows harshly. We spent a weekend there doing nothing but eating, drinking, talking, and walking on the beach. I think that was the most _hyggelig_ weekend I spent all year.

CASUALNESS

Most *hyggelige* moments seem to be built on a foundation of casualness. In order for you and your guests to be able to hygge, you need to feel relaxed. There is no need to make things formal. Come as you are and be as you are.

When I was in my twenties, I took part in the harvest of grapes one autumn in Champagne. A couple of years ago, I was visiting the region with three friends and we decided to stop by the Marquette vineyard where I had worked. We met Glennie, the lady of the house, and her son, who was by now a fully grown man, and spent a *hyggelig* afternoon at the vineyard and in the rustic country kitchen, with its low ceiling and flagstones, drinking wine at one of the long tables. The mood of the evening was relaxed and casual; despite the fact that I hadn't seen Glennie and her son for a number of years, there was no need for any formality.

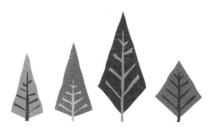

CLOSENESS TO NATURE

Whether you are sitting by a river in Sweden or in a vineyard in France, or just in your garden or nearby park, being surrounded by nature enables you to bring your guard down and adds a certain simplicity.

When we are close to nature, we are not engulfed in entertaining electronics or juggling a broad spectrum of options. There are no luxuries or extravagance, just good company and good conversation. Simple, slow, rustic elements are a fast track to hygge.

One summer I went camping with a group of friends along the Nissan River in Sweden. We were roasting chickens over the fire, and they were slowly turning nice and golden. In the fire, you could hear the sizzling of the baking potatoes wrapped in foil. We had paddled a fair distance in the canoes that day, and now darkness was falling. The fire lit up the trees surrounding our camp with warm colors, but despite the light from the fire, you could still see the stars through the treetops. As we waited for the golden chickens to be ready, we drank whiskey out of coffee mugs. We were silent, tired, and happy, and it was pure hygge.

BEING IN THE PRESENT MOMENT

There is an element of being present in those moments. Hygge is charged with a strong orientation and commitment toward experiencing and savoring the present moment.

On that camping trip, there was nowhere else we needed to be. We were off-line. No phone. No e-mail. We were surrounded by nature and good company, and were able to fully relax and take in the moment.

Every summer I go sailing with one of my best friends and his dad. There are few things I enjoy more than standing at the helm under full white sails and a blue sky, listening to the music blasting from below deck. The most *hyggelige* moments on these trips are when we are docked at the various harbors we visit. After every dinner we sit together and watch the sun set from the deck, while we listen to the wind in the rigging of the ships in the harbor and sip our post-dinner Irish coffee. That is hygge.

Creating hygge moments may be best achieved by using some of the elements mentioned above. Sometimes you may be able to get all the ingredients in the pot. For me, that happens in summer cabins. In many ways, life in a cabin offers all of the above, and all my favorite childhood memories gravitate toward a small summer cabin my family owned just six miles outside the city, where we would live from May to September. At that time of year, when even the night knows no darkness, my brother and I would enjoy endless days of summer. We would climb trees, catch fish, play football, ride bicycles, explore tunnels, sleep in tree houses, hide under boats on the beach, build dams and forts, play with bows and arrows, and search the forest for berries and hidden Nazi gold.

The cabin was a third of the size of our house in the city, the furniture was old, and the TV was black and white and had a fourteen-inch screen and a moody antenna. But this was the place where we had the most hygge. In many ways, these were the happiest times, and the most *hyggelige*. I think it may be because, in many ways, cabins include all the drivers of hygge: the smells, the sounds, and the simplicity. When you stay in one, there is a closer connection to nature and to each other. A cabin forces you to live more simply and slowly. To get out. To get together. To enjoy the moment.

HYGGE DURING OFFICE HOURS

However, hygge is not restricted to cozy cabins, Irish coffees on the deck, or snuggling up in your hyggekrog *at home in front of the fire. Danes believe that hygge can—and should—happen at the office.*

Exhibit A in this theory is, of course, the cake discussed in chapter 4. In addition, according to a survey on hygge conducted by the Happiness Research Institute, there is the evidence that 78 percent of Danes say that work should be *hyggeligt*, too.

Should it be *hyggeligt* to work?

78%
Yes

13%
No

9%
Don't Know

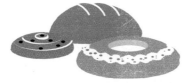

So, how do you make office hours more hyggeligt? Well, cakes and candles, obviously. But this is just the start. Think of ways to make things more casual, cozy, and egalitarian. Here are five ideas to get the hygge going at the office.

1. ORGANIZE A POTLUCK FRIDAY.

Instead of bringing lunch just for yourself, why not organize potlucks for lunch one day of the week? When everybody shares, everybody gets hygge.

2. SET UP AN OFFICE GARDEN.

If the office or the surroundings allow it, you can add to the hygge by planting a few plants. Spending a few minutes each day tending to them may be a nice way to manage stress. Extra hygge points if you grow produce that can be enjoyed at lunch.

3. BRING YOUR DOG TO WORK.

A few years ago, Michael, one of my interns had to take care of his mother's dog, Leica, for a few weeks and asked whether he could bring her to the office. Best weeks ever. Having Leica at the office definitely increased the hygge and office joy. I made a deal with myself that after accomplishing an item on my to-do list, I could go and pet Leica. My productivity went through the roof.

4. TRY TO MAKE THE OFFICE MORE HOMEY.

Could we put in a couple of couches for people to use when they have long reports to read or need to hold a quick and informal meeting? I do a lot of interviews because of my work and I prefer sitting on the couch with the journalist and having a good conversation with them, instead of the two of us facing each other across a fancy table in a sterile office setting.

5. HYGGE CUBICLE LIFE.

Maybe you can't change the office, but what about your desk? Could you add some plants, have some hygge socks in the drawer for working in the late evenings? Or go all the way, think of your cubicle as the Batcave of hygge and be the secret hygge hero at the office. The one that leaves a nice piece of chocolate at your colleagues' desks while they are at lunch.

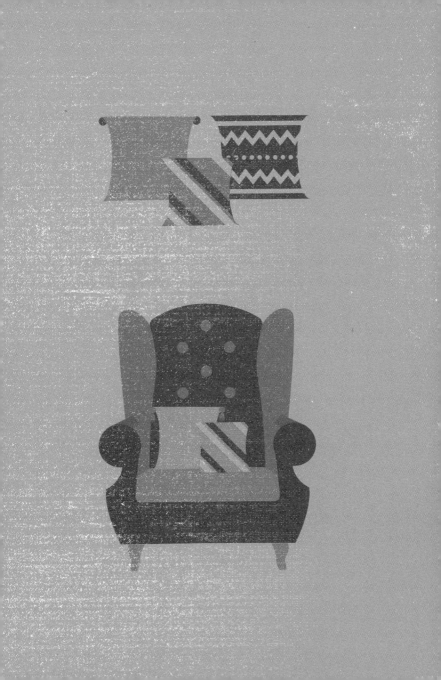

CHAPTER EIGHT

HYGGE ALL YEAR ROUND

NOT JUST FOR CHRISTMAS

In Denmark, a popular saying goes "There is no bad weather, only bad clothing." But, frankly, there are not a lot of great things to say about the weather in Denmark.

Some describe the Danish weather as dark, windy, and damp; some say Denmark has two winters, one gray and one green.

With this kind of weather, it will come as no surprise that Danes spend most of their time indoors in the winter months.

In summertime, most Danes spend as much time as possible outside, desperately hoping to enjoy some sun, but in the months from November to March, the weather forces Danes to stay indoors. As Danes do not have the opportunity to enjoy winter activities in their own country, as in Sweden and Norway, or to spend time outdoors in the winter period, as in southern Europe, all Danes have left to do is hygge at home. As a result, the high season for hygge is autumn and winter, according to a study on hygge conducted by the Happiness Research Institute.

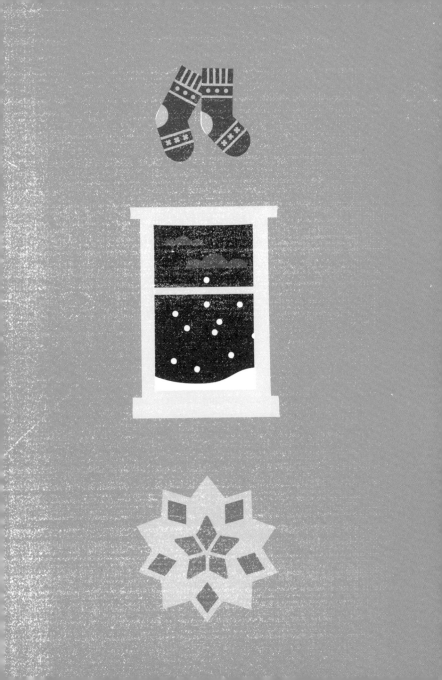

Here is a selection of ideas for how to hygge throughout the year.

JANUARY: MOVIE NIGHT

The month of January is the perfect time to relax with friends and family with a casual movie night. Let each person bring snacks to share, and pick out one of the old classics, one that you've all seen, so it doesn't matter too much if people chat a bit during the film.

An entertaining add-on to movie night is to come up with the shortest way of explaining the plot of the given movie. This turns *The Lord of the Rings* trilogy into "Group spends nine hours returning jewelry" and *Forrest Gump* into "Drug-addicted girl takes advantage of mentally challenged boy for decades."

FEBRUARY: SKI TRIP

If you have the opportunity, organize your friends and family to head to the mountains at this time of the year. Yes, the view in the mountains is stunning, the speed on the slopes is exhilarating, and the purity of the air is amazing—but the best part of the ski trip is the hygge. The magic happens when you and your crew get back to your cabin, tired from the slopes, dirty, and messy-haired, and relax with coffee in shared silence. Remember to pack the Grand Marnier!

MARCH: THEME MONTH

If you and your family are going somewhere on vacation in the summer this might be a way to get a jump on the hygge. If you are going to Spain, spend March exploring the country from afar. By "exploring," I mean watch Spanish movies, make tapas, and if you have kids, maybe spend one evening putting Post-its on the chairs (*sillas*), table (*mesa*), plates (*platos*) in Spanish, so you can get a head start with the language. If you are not going on vacation this year, you can either take the theme from a country you have been to previously (get those photo albums out) or pick your dream destination. If you can't go to the country, bring the country home to you.

APRIL: HIKING AND COOKING OVER AN OPEN FIRE

April can be a wonderful month to go hiking, camping, or canoeing. Weather-wise, it may be a bit brisk, so remember to pack those woolen socks (they are extra *hyggelige*), but the month offers benefits in terms of fewer mosquitoes. If you are a city dweller like me, it is natural to panic in the first hours of a hike, thinking, "What the hell will we do out here without Wi-Fi?" However, once you overcome this, your heart rate and stress levels will drop. Hiking is an Easter egg of hygge, as it includes slowness, rusticity, and togetherness. Gather the wood, build the fire, prepare the food, and watch it cook slowly over the fire, then enjoy the after-dinner whiskey with your friends under the stars.

Remember to pack the chocolate eggs for the kids if you are heading out for Easter.

MAY: WEEKEND CABIN

The days are getting longer, and May is the time to start making use of the countryside. One of your friends might have access to a cabin, or you may find a cheap rental—the more rustic the cabin, the more hygge. A fireplace is a bonus. Be sure to pack board games for rainy afternoons. A weekend in May might also present the first opportunity of the year for a barbecue. In terms of summer hygge, nothing beats standing around the grill with a beer in your hand.

JUNE: ELDERFLOWER CORDIAL AND THE SUMMER SOLSTICE

Early June is the perfect time to harvest elderflowers to make cordial or lemonade.

St John's Eve falls on June 23, and on that evening Danes celebrate the summer solstice. This is my favorite tradition. In Denmark, the sun in June sets close to 11 p.m. on a night that never lets go of the light completely. As the sun sets, there is a bittersweet acknowledgment that, from tomorrow, we will start the slow descent into darkness as the days shorten. This is the perfect evening for a picnic. Grab your friends and family and light a bonfire. (They are usually lit relatively late because of the light, so if you need to entertain the kids during the wait, this is a great evening for an egg-and-spoon race.)

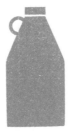

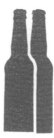

ELDERFLOWER CORDIAL

Whether you drink it cold on a hot summer
day or warm during winter, this elderflower cordial will
have the smell of summer. And not only when you drink it:
to make the cordial you have to leave the flowers and the
lemons in a pan for twenty-four hours, so your whole house
will smell of summer hygge. Just one whiff immediately
transports me back to my childhood summers.

For 10½ cups of elderflower lemonade, serves 10–12

30 elderflower clusters

3 large lemons

6 cups water

8 cups sugar

1. Wash elderflower clusters well and place them in a large bowl.

2. Scrub the lemons under hot water, slice them, and add them to
   the clusters in the bowl.

3. Bring the water to a boil and add the sugar.

4. Pour the hot water into the bowl containing the elderflower clusters and lemon slices.

5. Cover the bowl with a lid and let the lemonade rest for three days.

6. Strain the liquid and pour it into bottles. Store in the fridge.

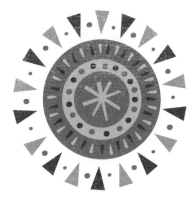

JULY: SUMMER PICNIC

July is when Danes really love to get out and enjoy nature. The weather is warm and the evenings are still long. This is the perfect time of year for a picnic by the sea, in a meadow, or in a park. The choice is yours, but get out of town. Invite your family, friends, neighbors, or the people who just moved in down the street. Make it a potluck event, so everybody brings a dish or two to share. Potluck dinners are usually more *hyggelig*, because they are more egalitarian. They are about sharing food and sharing the responsibility and chores.

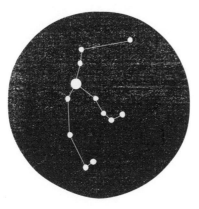

AUGUST: THE PERSEID METEOR SHOWER

Bring blankets for a night under the stars. While the light nights at this time of year may not be the best in which to watch stars, the Perseid meteor shower occurs in mid-August, usually reaching peak activity around the eleventh to the thirteenth. Look northeast for the Perseus constellation, which has Andromeda to the east and Cassiopeia to the north. If you have kids, this is a great time to bring a book of stories from Greek mythology to read while you wait for the shooting stars.

For people in the southern hemisphere, the Eta Aquarid meteor shower is an option. It usually peaks between late April and mid-May.

SEPTEMBER: MUSHROOM FORAGING

Mushrooms appear mainly in the autumn but can be found from late summer on. There is no better taste than food you have grown, caught, or foraged yourself—and it has a high hygge factor. Bring family and friends for a forage excursion to the forest.

WARNING: Eating the wrong sort of mushrooms can be deadly, so find an experienced mushroom forager and ask them to come along on a forage. Many communities organize group tours.

OCTOBER: CHESTNUTS

It is chestnut season. If you have kids, take them chestnut hunting and use the chestnuts to make animal figurines.

For the adults, buy edible chestnuts, make a cross with a knife in the pointy end, and roast them in the oven at 200 degrees for about thirty minutes, until the skins open and the insides are tender. Peel off the tough outside skin and add a bit of butter and salt.

If you just want quality hygge time by yourself, pick up some mandarins, roasted chestnuts, and a copy of *A Moveable Feast* by Hemingway. It is set in 1920s Paris, when Hemingway was working as a penniless writer.

NOVEMBER: SOUP COOK-OFF

Winter is coming. It is time to get out the old soup recipes and find new ones. Invite family and friends over for a soup cook-off. Each person brings ingredients for a soup to feed one person. Take turns preparing small dishes of different soups, enough for everyone to try. I usually make a pumpkin-ginger soup, which works really well with a bit of crème fraîche. If you want to do something extra as host, bake some homemade bread. The smell of freshly baked bread is definitely hygge.

DECEMBER: *GLØGG* AND *ÆBLESKIVER* (PANCAKE PUFFS)

This is hygge high season. The consumption of candles and confectionery soars, as do BMIs. This is also prime time for *gløgg* (you'll find the recipe on page 74). Start out well in advance by soaking those raisins in port and invite your friends and family over for an afternoon or evening of *gløgg* and *æbleskiver* (recipe on page 176).

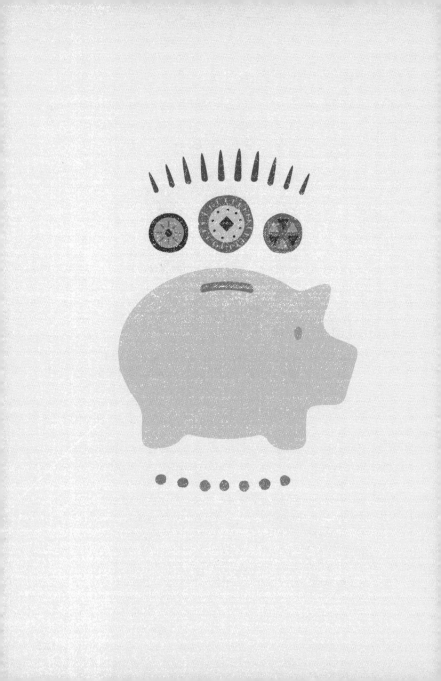

—

CHAPTER NINE

HYGGE ON THE CHEAP

THE BEST THINGS IN LIFE ARE FREE

There is nothing fancy, expensive, or luxurious about a pair of ugly woolen hygge socks—and that is a vital feature of the anatomy of hygge. Champagne and oysters may be many things, but hygge is not one of them.

Hygge is humble and slow. It is choosing rustic over new, simple over posh and ambience over excitement. In many ways, hygge might be the Danish cousin to slow and simple living.

It is wearing your pajamas and watching *Lord of the Rings* the day before Christmas, it is sitting in your window watching the weather while sipping your favorite tea, and it is looking into the bonfire on summer solstice surrounded by your friends and family while your twistbread slowly bakes.

Simplicity and modesty are central to hygge, but they are also considered virtues when it comes to Danish design and culture. Simplicity and functionality are the main ingredients of Danish design classics, and the Danes' love affair with modesty means that bragging about your accomplishments and flashing your Rolex are not only frowned upon and considered poor taste, but spoil the hygge. In short, the more bling, the less hygge.

Consequently, you can also play the hygge card as an exit strategy if you enter a high-end restaurant you can't afford. "Shouldn't we find a place that is more *hyggeligt*?" is a perfectly valid reason to find a cheaper establishment. Not Noma, though. That restaurant is really *hyggeligt*. It has the right lighting.

Hygge is about appreciating the simple pleasures in life and can be achieved on a shoestring budget. The poem and song "The Happy Day of Svante" by Benny Andersen is famous in Denmark. It's all about savoring the moment and enjoying simple pleasures: "Look, real daylight soon. Red sun and waning moon. She takes a shower for me. Me whom it's good to be. Life's not bad, for it's all we have got. And the coffee's almost hot."

Okay, so Danes might be better at hygge than poetry, but one of the most consistent patterns in happiness research is how little difference money makes. Of course, if you can't afford to eat, money is of the utmost importance, but if you're not battling poverty or struggling to make ends meet, an additional $100 per month is not going to move the needle when it comes to happiness.

This fits well with hygge. You cannot buy the right atmosphere or a sense of togetherness. You cannot hygge if you are in a hurry or stressed out, and the art of creating intimacy cannot be bought by anything but time, interest, and engagement in the people around you.

Hygge can and often will be about eating or drinking, but the more it counteracts consumption, the more *hyggeligt* it is. The more money and prestige is associated with something, the less *hyggeligt* it becomes. The simpler and more primitive an activity is, the more *hyggeligt* it is. Drinking tea is more *hyggeligt* than drinking champagne, playing board games is more *hyggeligt* than playing computer games, and home-cooked food and biscuits are more *hyggeligt* than store-bought ones.

In short, if you want hygge, there is no amount of money that you can spend which will increase the hygge factor—at least not if you are buying anything more expensive than a candle. Hygge is an atmosphere that is not only unimproved by spending more money on it, but rather, in some ways, the opposite.

Hygge may be bad fort capitalism, but it may prove to be very good for your personal happiness. Hygge is appreciating the simple pleasures in life and can be achieved with very little money. Here are ten examples how the best hygge in life is free—or almost so.

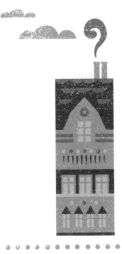

TEN INEXPENSIVE HYGGE ACTIVITIES

---

1. BRING OUT THE BOARD GAMES

We live in the age of Netflix, Candy Crush, and an endless supply of electronic entertainment. We hang out with technology instead of with each other. However, playing board games is still popular—in part because of the hygge. Every year, my friend Martin organizes the mother of board games: a game of Axis & Allies. Set in World War II, it is essentially a complex version of the game Risk. The game usually lasts for about fourteen hours, and Martin usually leaves his very understanding girlfriend in a hotel for the night. We make the evening into more than simply playing a game. There'll be classical music on—mostly Wagner and Beethoven—and smoke from cigars fills the room, so you can barely see our group of grown men in uniforms. Admittedly, we may take it to an extreme level, but we do it for the hygge.

But why are board games hygge? Well, first of all, it is a social activity. You play games together. You create common memories and strengthen bonds. All of Martin's friends still remember the moment in the 2012 game when the Allies suddenly realized that Moscow would fall. In addition, for many of us who grew up with Monopoly or Trivial Pursuit, board games are full of nostalgia and take us back to simpler times. There is also a slowness to the activity (especially if the game takes fourteen hours), a tangibility, and an air of hygge.

2. PANTRY PARTY

This is one of my favorites. Invite your friends over to your house for an afternoon or an evening of cooking and hygge. The rules are simple. Every person brings ingredients to make something that goes in the pantry (or in the fridge). Strawberry jam, sweet pickle relish, ketchup, chicken stock, limoncello, pumpkin soup—you name it. Everybody also brings jars, cans, bottles, or containers in a shape that will allow them to store a bounty of homemade treats. The beauty of it is the diversity. Instead of having ten servings of pumpkin soup, you now have mango chutney, ginger beer, pickled chili, baba ghanoush, a loaf of sourdough bread, plum marmalade, elderflower cordial, walnut aquavit, and raspberry sorbet. Yum.

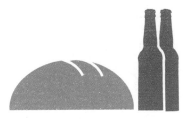

3. TV NIGHT

One of my best friends and I always watch *Game of Thrones* together. Every two weeks or so, we watch two episodes. No more. I know it is borderline Amish in the age of Netflix not to binge-watch a whole season of your favorite show once it is released, but this approach has some advantages. First, it brings TV back to being something more sociable. Second, it allows you to look forward to something on a regular basis. So restrain yourself from bingeing and invite friends over for weekly viewings of a specific TV show.

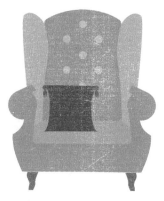

4. CROQUET

Playing croquet is a great way of hanging out with family and friends. The game is informal and slow, so it allows for conversation at the same time and there is something to watch while you talk. Find the nearest park or a yard with a stretch of grass you can use as a croquet field, and bring blankets and a picnic basket.

5. SET UP A MINI-LIBRARY

An inexpensive and sustainable way to make a shared space (in your apartment building or neighborhood) a little bit more *hyggeligt* is to build a small library. Find a rustic dresser or some shelves and put them in the hallway or on the stairway landing (you may want to ask for permission first). Put a handful or more of the books you have already read in the library, but let your neighbors help you increase the selection of titles by following the principle of leaving a book whenever you take one. Being greeted with a display of books when you come into your building is a more *hyggelig* way of returning home. Also, it may encourage more hygge interaction among the tenants.

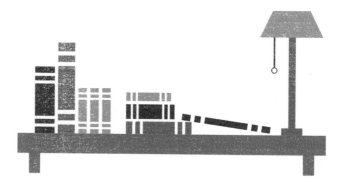

6. MAKE A FIRE

A fire is definitely part of the hygge equation and so is the slow preparation of very unfussy food, but also involved is the togetherness around the fire, the fact that there is no need to keep the conversation going because you have the sound of the fire. Now the fire has burned down and the embers are ready. You have found a suitable straight stick and stripped the bark from the end. Wrap the bread tightly around the stick and place it over the glowing embers. People are gathered in a close circle around the fire now, moving around a little as the smoke changes direction. Your eyes hurt from the smoke, your hand hurts from being close to the fire, and your bread is turning black on the outside yet remaining unbaked on the inside. But it doesn't get any more *hyggelig* than this.

7. OUTDOOR MOVIES

Many cities offer outdoor film screenings during the summer. In Copenhagen, they take place during August, as in June and July it is simply too bright in the evenings to show movies. The sound is usually difficult to hear, you sit kind of uncomfortably on the ground, without back support, and the people who were smart enough to bring small chairs set up camp right in front of you and thus block some of your view of the screen. However, it is still total *hyggeligt*. I often go with a couple of friends. We set up camp, eat some food, drink some wine, talk, and wait for the movie to start.

8. SWAP PARTY

Remember that lamp you have in your basement and have been meaning to put on eBay for two years now? Or that extra blender you and your partner now have since you decided to move in together? Why not get rid of it by swapping it for something that you do need—and have a *hyggelig* evening at the same time? Invite friends and family over for a swap party. The rules are simple. Each person brings something he or she doesn't use anymore that could be of value to someone else. Beyond being wallet- and eco-friendly, it is also a nice opportunity to clean out your wardrobe, kitchen cabinet, basement, or wherever you store the things you never use. Furthermore, it may be more convenient and fun to swap with friends than to spend a weekend pushing your junk at the flea market or posting a listing.

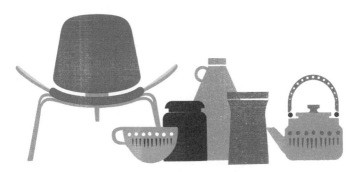

9. SLEDDING

In the wintertime, it is easy to feel stuck inside. And while it can be *hyggeligt* to relax with your book and a cup of tea, it is even more *hyggeligt* after you have spent a day in the snow. So gather a group of people and head for the hills. If you have a beautiful wooden sleigh stashed in the basement, great, but cheaper options exist. You can use a sturdy plastic bag to sleigh down a hill. Sledding is free and fun. Bring a winter picnic basket with tea or mulled wine for afterward. Don't drink and sled.

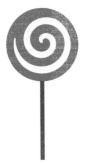

10. PLAY

In many ways, some of the activities above, like sledding and board games, fall into the same category—play. We loved them when we were kids but for some reason we stop doing them when we become grown-ups. Adults are not supposed to play. We are supposed to stress, worry, and be too busy dealing with life's problems. But according to a study undertaken by Princeton University and led by Alan Krueger, professor in economics and public affairs there, we are happiest when we are involved in engaging leisure activities.

One of our issues as adults is that we become too focused on the results of an activity. We work to earn money. We go to the gym to lose weight. We spend time with people to network and further our careers. What happened to doing something just because it's fun? Notice in the table (on pages 152–53) how social activities such as sports, hiking, partying, and playing with children are the top scorers.

THE PRINCETON AFFECT AND TIME SURVEY

In this study, around 4,000 respondents were asked how happy the different activities they had engaged in during the day before had made them feel, on a scale of 0 to 6.

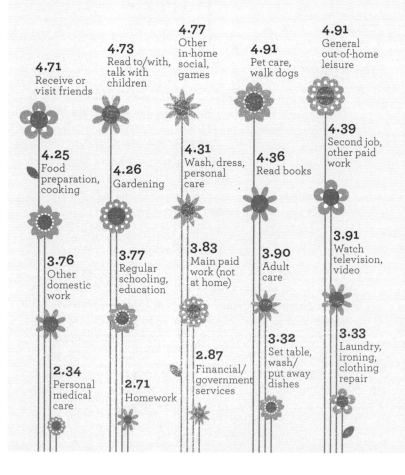

4.71 Receive or visit friends

4.73 Read to/with, talk with children

4.77 Other in-home social, games

4.91 Pet care, walk dogs

4.91 General out-of-home leisure

4.39 Second job, other paid work

4.25 Food preparation, cooking

4.26 Gardening

4.31 Wash, dress, personal care

4.36 Read books

3.76 Other domestic work

3.77 Regular schooling, education

3.83 Main paid work (not at home)

3.90 Adult care

3.91 Watch television, video

2.34 Personal medical care

2.71 Homework

2.87 Financial/government services

3.32 Set table, wash/put away dishes

3.33 Laundry, ironing, clothing repair

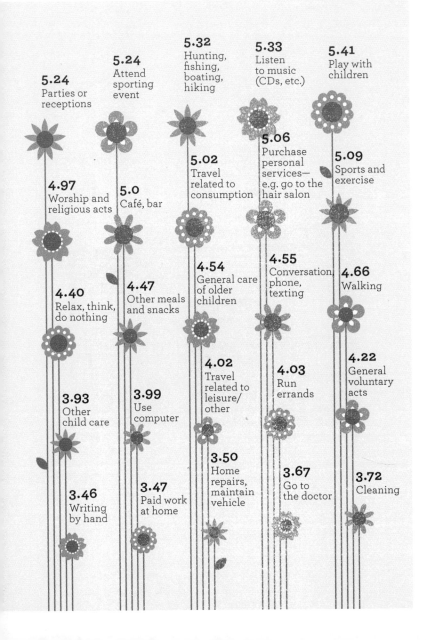

5.24
Parties or receptions

5.24
Attend sporting event

5.32
Hunting, fishing, boating, hiking

5.33
Listen to music (CDs, etc.)

5.41
Play with children

5.06
Purchase personal services— e.g. go to the hair salon

5.09
Sports and exercise

5.02
Travel related to consumption

4.97
Worship and religious acts

5.0
Café, bar

4.55
Conversation, phone, texting

4.66
Walking

4.54
General care of older children

4.40
Relax, think, do nothing

4.47
Other meals and snacks

4.22
General voluntary acts

4.02
Travel related to leisure/ other

4.03
Run errands

3.93
Other child care

3.99
Use computer

3.72
Cleaning

3.50
Home repairs, maintain vehicle

3.67
Go to the doctor

3.46
Writing by hand

3.47
Paid work at home

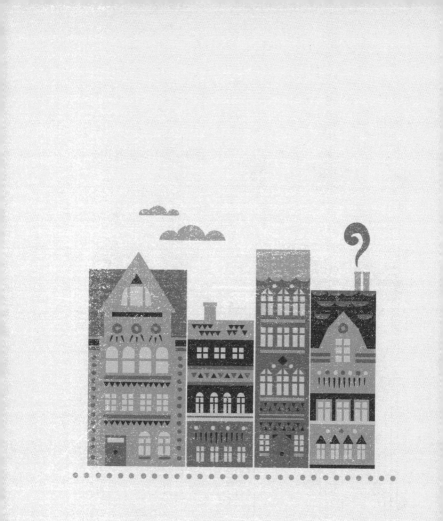

———

CHAPTER TEN

HYGGE TOUR OF COPENHAGEN

HYGGE SAFARI

If you should visit Copenhagen, you might want to visit some of these hyggelige *places.*

NYHAVN (NEW HARBOR)

This used to be a dodgy part of town with rowdy sailors and "ladies of pleasure." Today you can visit one of the many restaurants for a pickled herring and schnapps. If that is not your thing, and if the weather is nice, do like the locals and buy a few beers from a shop, have a seat at the bulwark, and watch the city go by.

LA GLACE

Dive into the cream. Remember the importance of cakes? If there were a Camino de Santiago for cake, La Glace would be the Santiago de Compostela Cathedral. La Glace was established in 1870 and is the oldest confectionery shop in Denmark.

TIVOLI GARDENS

The Tivoli Gardens were founded in 1843 and are a classic attraction in Copenhagen, where many citizens purchase annual passes to the gardens. While many people visit during the summer, the best time for hygge is when Tivoli dresses up for Christmas and New Year's Eve (usually from mid-November until January). This is a celebration of light. Several hundred thousand lights turn the garden into a magical place in the winter darkness, and you can enjoy some *gløgg* near one of the bonfires in the garden or get warm by the fireplace at Nimb Bar.

ROWBOAT IN CHRISTIANSHAVN

Christianshavn is part of the city center in Copenhagen but it is separated from the rest of the center by the Inner Harbor. It is dominated by canals and may remind you a little of Amsterdam. The best way to experience this part of town is by renting a rowboat and rowing along the canals. Bring blankets, wine, and a picnic basket.

GRÅBRØDRETORV

Being surrounded by the old houses here will transport you back centuries. This *hyggelige* square gets its name from the monastery of the Grey Brothers (*Grå brødre*), established in 1238. There are plenty of cozy restaurants in the square. At Peder Oxe you can get classical Danish *smørrebrød* and enjoy the fireplace. Even one of the hairdressing salons has a fireplace (and a French bulldog, who will happily sleep on your lap while you have your hair cut). Total hygge. You might also be lucky enough to see a full pig roast at the square.

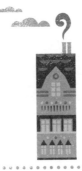

VÆRNEDAMSVEJ

At Værnedamsvej, cars zigzag between cyclists and pedestrians. This short street will make you slow down and smell the flowers and the coffee. Florists, cafés, wine bars, and interior design shops make this a wonderful place to spend a lazy and *hyggelig* afternoon.

A *SMØRREBRØD* PLACE

Smørrebrød means, literally, spread bread. It is an open sandwich on rye bread. Danes are huge fans of rye bread, so it is usually one of the first things they miss when they are living abroad. Some expats living in Denmark will, however, refer to the bread as the devil's sandals, as they really dislike the taste and find the bread tough to chew. In all regards, *smørrebrød* is a truly Danish lunch experience. *Smørrebrød* can have an almost limitless number of toppings, from herring to raw beef, egg, and seafood, and some have colorful names like "the veterinarian's night food." *Smørrebrød* is usually served with beer and schnapps. In Copenhagen, you will find many traditional *smørrebrød* places, and such a lunch will surely get the hygge going.

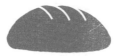

LIBRARY BAR

In the Plaza Hotel, near the central train station, you will find the Library Bar, which opened in 1914. Here are sofas, wooden panels, leather-bound books, and really *hyggelig* lighting. The bar features live music from time to time, but on a quiet night it is well suited for deep conversation. If you visit during Christmas, you will find a Christmas tree hanging upside down from the ceiling.

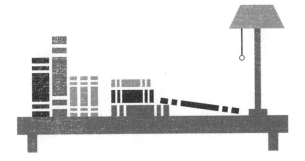

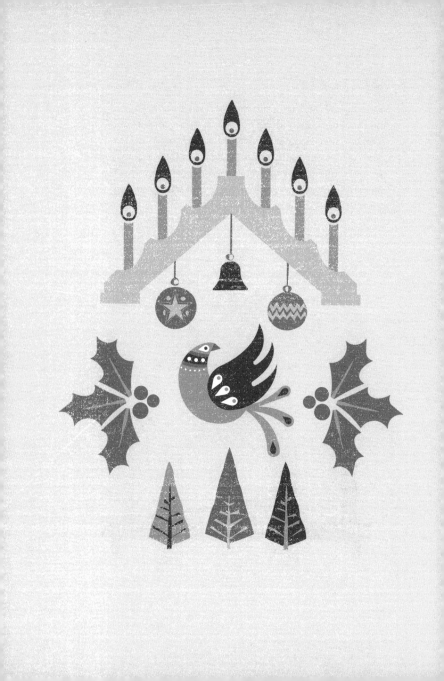

CHAPTER ELEVEN

—

CHRISTMAS

IT'S THE MOST *HYGGELIG* TIME OF YEAR

———

For many people—Danes included—Christmas is a wonderful time. However, wonderful is far from the only word used to describe it. If you ask people of any nationality to describe Christmas in one word, adjectives like happy, cheerful, warm, *and* heartfelt *would probably surface. Danes would agree with a lot of these. But, they would object, "the most fitting word is missing. You forgot* hyggelig!"

In Denmark, in one month of the year, the days are so short you will be lucky to catch a glimpse of the sun. Riding your bike to and from work in the cold and wet and in complete darkness, you begin to question why anybody ever thought that settling in Denmark would be a good idea. Yes, I know, in Denmark it is not –30 degrees outside, nor are we troubled with hurricanes or tsunamis. But living here, you do get the sense that the weather gods have taken a certain disliking to the Danes; that they want us to feel miserable and uncomfortable at least one month a year.

As unlikely as it sounds, this is the season of hygge in Denmark. Danes simply will not let the weather or the laws of nature define their emotional well-being. Therefore, instead of going into hibernation—which does indeed seem appealing on damp December mornings—Danes have decided to make the best of things.

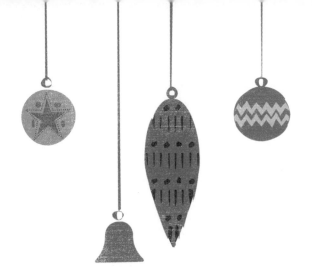

Even though it is possible to hygge all year round, only once a year is hygge the ultimate goal of an entire month. Without achieving hygge, a Dane's toil for the Christmas project is redundant. Chestnuts, a fireplace, friends, and family coming together around a table of delicious treats; decorations of red, green, and gold; the fresh scent of pine from the Christmas tree; carols everybody knows; and the broadcasting of the very same TV shows as last year—and every year before that—these are features of a fairly ordinary Christmas all over the world. From Dallas to Durban, people sing along to the words of "Last Christmas." From Dublin to Dubai, people know the plot of *A Christmas Carol.* This is no less true in Denmark.

Indeed, there are Christmas traditions which are specifically Danish, but a Danish Christmas is not considerably different from a German, French, or British one in terms of activities or traditions.

What is different in Denmark, though, is that a Danish Christmas will always be planned, thought of, and evaluated in relation to the concept of hygge. At no other time of the year will you hear Danes mentioning hygge as much. It is literally mentioned at any given opportunity. And, of course, Danish includes a compound word, *julehygge* (Christmas hygge), which is both an adjective and a verb. "Do you want to come over for some *julehygge*?"

In the pages that follow, I will try to outline a recipe for a proper *hyggelig* Christmas—a perfect Danish Christmas—which is in itself a daunting task. Danes hold their Christmas dear, and I am sure a lot of Danes will disagree with the elements of Christmas I am going to mention. However, most will probably recognize more than one element from their own traditions.

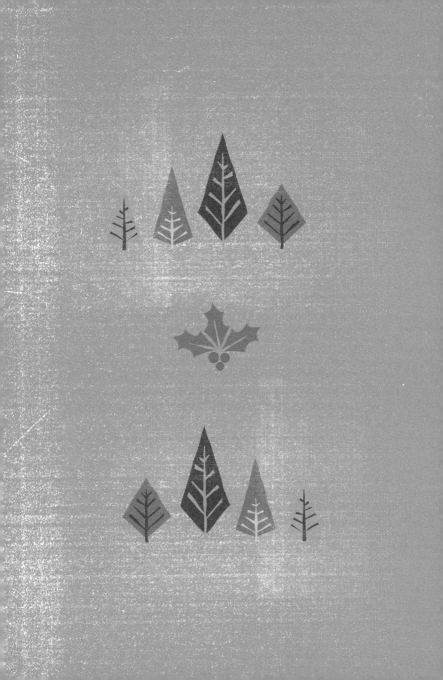

FAMILY AND FRIENDS

Every year in the second half of December, a full-blown migration takes place in Denmark. People originally from other parts of Denmark who usually live in Copenhagen pack their stuff, plus tons of presents, and jump on a train headed toward their hometown.

A *hyggelig* Christmas begins and ends with family and friends. Those are the people we feel safe around, the ones who make us feel comfortable. They know us, and we enjoy spending time with them because we love them. Time and time again, the quality of our social relations has been shown to be one of the best predictors for our emotional well-being.

In our everyday lives, many of us feel we see too little of our loved ones. Christmas is an opportunity to make up for that; to gather around a table full of delicious treats in order to enjoy life and one another's company. That is the key ingredient in a *hyggelig* Christmas. People all over the world do the very same each year, but only in Danish homes do people draw a collective sigh of relief when someone reassures the others that "This is *hyggeligt*." In that moment, both hosts and guests feel that Christmas has arrived; the proper spirit of hygge has been achieved.

But family is not enough in order to put together a *hyggelig* Christmas. Even though a lot of people see friends and family mostly during the holidays, this can be done all year round.

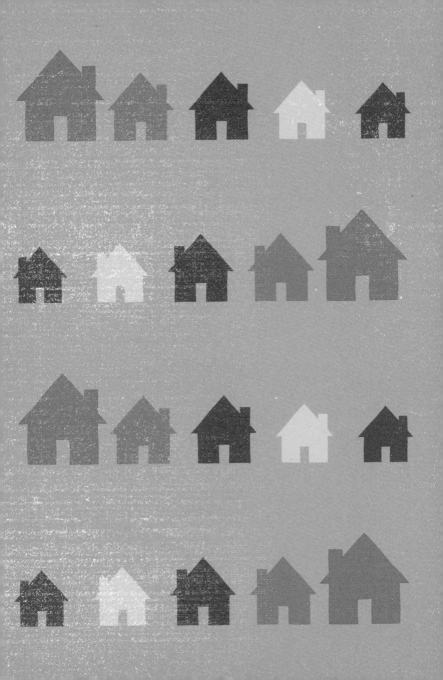

TRADITIONS

FOOD

Around Christmastime, certain rituals and traditions must be adhered to in order to achieve hygge. A Danish Christmas needs the proper decorations, food, and activities in order to be considered a "real" *hyggelig* Christmas.

First, there is the food. Danish food. Heavy Danish food. If you search the Internet for long enough, I am convinced you will find diets that include almost everything. There are diets where you eat only meat or only fat, water diets, diets with lots of carbs and diets without any. There are diets of vegetables and even diets of sunlight. Nonetheless, I have yet to come across a diet that would accept Danish Christmas food.

The main protagonist in the Christmas menu is the meat, which is either roast pork or duck—often both. It will be accompanied by boiled potatoes, or caramelized potatoes, stewed sweet-and-sour red cabbage, gravy, and pickled gherkins. Some have cream-stewed cabbage, sausages, and various types of bread, too.

To complete the feast, we have a truly Danish invention: *risalamande* (it comes from the French *ris à l'amande*, and this makes it sound fancier) is half part-whipped cream, half part-boiled rice, with finely chopped almonds and topped with hot cherry sauce. Eating *risalamande* is not just a delicious experience, though. It is very much social. Because hidden in the big bowl of dessert is one whole almond.

Usually, when everybody has been served a bowl of *risalamande*, a silence spreads across the room. Eyes shift from person to person. It is more similar to a poker game or a Western-style shootout than a Christmas tradition. "Who's got the almond?" Whoever finds it gets a present and will be the subject of comments about always being lucky (and, somehow it does actually seem that some people are better at getting the almond than others).

Soon the silence is replaced by questions: "You've got the almond, haven't you?," "You're hiding it, just like last year, aren't you?" The aim of the one who has found the almond is to hide it and deny having found it in order to lure the others into eating everything in their bowl: it becomes a kind of perverted eating contest. Around Christmastime, eating a dessert turns into a *hyggelig* social activity in itself. Do you think it sounds delicious? You should taste it. Fortunately for our bodies, we only get to feast on these dishes once a year.

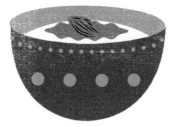

DECORATIONS

No *hyggelig* Christmas is complete without the proper decorations. These may vary even more than the food, as every family has inherited its own decorations from parents and grandparents. But they may include figures of *nisse* (an elf or gnome), animals, and Father Christmas, mini-nativity figures and cornets or woven hearts made of glossy paper.

Woven paper hearts are rarely seen outside Denmark. Their origin has been attributed to Hans Christian Andersen, who was a master at paper cuttings. They're made out of two double-layered cutouts of glossy paper, and the flaps of the two cutouts are woven together to make the heart shape. They come in various colors and have different motifs, and every Dane knows how to craft at least a simple one. (See page 179 for instructions on how to make your own woven hearts.)

Then there are candles (of course). When 100 percent of the time spent at home in December is during the hours of darkness, you need various sources of lighting, and candles are *hyggelige*. A specific Danish version of a Christmas candle is the advent candle, painted like a tape measure with dates from December 1 to December 24.

Each day the corresponding piece of candle is burned away. However, few people light the calendar candle when they are on their own. Rather, it is done either in the morning, when parents are frantically trying to get everybody ready for school and work, or in the evening, when darkness has spread again and the family is assembled around the dinner table. The calendar light is literally the centerpiece of the family. It constitutes a natural point and time marker to assemble around. And besides, it feeds the Danes' fetish for the countdown to Christmas.

COUNTDOWN TO HYGGE

The advent candle is not the only way Danes count down to the ultimate hygge day of the year. Danish children have advent calendars and open a flap each day to unveil a Christmas symbol or motif.

A more extravagant version is a series of boxes of wood or cardboard, each of which contains, say, a small Christmas bauble or a sweet. Some families even have present calendars and children get a small present each day until Christmas—when they will get even more.

And then there are the TV calendars. They are mostly for kids and provide a *hyggelig* activity to make their wait for the big day tolerable. Every year, most TV stations have their own *julekalender*—a story usually related to Christmas with twenty-four connected episodes, reaching a climax on December 24, when the adults are busy with last-minute preparations.

Emphasizing that Christmas really is the time for hygge, one of the recurring characters in these shows is Lunte, a *nisse*, who usually greets people by saying, "*Hyggehejsa*" (hygge hello). A new TV calendar is produced every year, and there is always an old one that is being shown again. And while children are laughing and having a good time watching these shows, you will often find the adults snatching glimpses of the screen and smiling to themselves, reminiscing about being a child and watching the very same scenes while waiting for the coming of Christmas Day.

Naturally, these things are in themselves *hyggelige*. But they are also important because they are traditions. And traditions matter to hygge. Traditions remind us of all the other good times we have had with family and friends. We feel there is a part of Christmas or hygge hidden in these actions and items that have been part of our whole life. Without them, something is missing. Christmas just would not be the same.

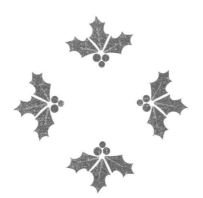

THE RACE TO RELAX

Getting a bit out of breath reading about all the necessities for a Danish Christmas? I completely get it. All the things I have sketched out here do contribute to the pressure for hygge around Christmas.

If people are not feeling the hygge, something is not right. Christmas is deemed a failure.

All the preparations for a *hyggelig* Christmas are quite often stressful and, indeed, not very *hyggelige*. Now, this may seem a bit contradictory, but it actually makes sense. Hygge is possible only if it stands in opposition to something which is not hygge. It is essential for the concept of hygge that it constitutes an alternative to everything that is not *hyggeligt* in our everyday lives. For a brief moment, hygge protects us against that which is not *hyggeligt*. There must be anti-hygge for hygge to be valuable. Life might seem stressful. It might seem unsafe and unfair. Life is often centered on money and social status. But life is none of these things in moments of hygge.

Remember my friend who commented that the only way our time in the cabin could be more *hyggelig* was if a storm broke outside? This is hygge. The more it sets the here and now apart from the tough realities of the outside world, the more valuable it becomes.

In this way, achieving hygge would not be possible without all the bustle and turmoil leading up to Christmas. All the money, stress, work, and time being sacrificed in the preparations for Christmas leads up to hygge as a climax. Hygge is postponed in order to be accomplished. Knowing friends and family have worked hard all December in order to get together and not focus on work, money, and all things profane is the meaning of hygge.

But Christmas still includes moments that threaten to compromise hygge. As hygge is about letting go of the everyday, the focus on, for example, money and the giving and exchanging of presents always threatens to contaminate the pure and pristine hygge.

Giving and receiving presents may cause someone to feel exposed or emphasize differences in status. Receiving too big a gift makes you feel in debt to the giver, while giving too big a gift is frowned upon, as it asserts the giver's superior position. Demonstrations of power are not welcome in hygge. In Denmark, Christmas hygge is egalitarian. It is about relations and community, not individuals trying to draw attention to themselves. It is not possible to achieve hygge if anybody feels excluded or superior to anybody else.

Therefore, the best Christmases are the ones where everything outlined in this chapter is achieved and where the danger element of gift-giving is eliminated by striking a balance between giving and receiving. Fortunately, once the presents have been exchanged, there are plenty of gift-free, *hyggelige* days of relaxation and lunches until New Year's Eve, when hygge is again sacrificed so that even more preparations can be made.

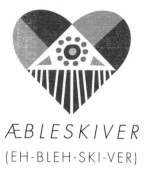

ÆBLESKIVER

(EH-BLEH-SKI-VER)

A traditional Danish treat for the Christmas
holidays is æbleskiver. Don't forget to serve it with gløgg—
(see the recipe for gløgg on page 74). For this you
need a special pan—an æbleskiver pan—which can
be found and ordered online.

Serves 4–6.

**Cooking time 45 minutes
(including 30 minutes rest for the dough)**

3 eggs

Scant 2 cups buttermilk

2 cups flour

1 tablespoon sugar

¼ teaspoon salt

½ teaspoon baking soda

3 tablespoons melted butter

confectioner's sugar, to serve

jam, to serve

1. Mix egg yolks, buttermilk, flour, sugar, salt, and baking soda together well. Cover the mixture and let it rest for thirty minutes.

2. Once the mixture has risen, whip the egg whites until stiff and fold gently into the mixture.

3. Heat the *æbleskiver* pan and put a little butter in each hole. Pour some of the mixture into each hole, filling them three-quarters full and cook over a medium heat. Turn the *æbleskiver* frequently, so they are cooked evenly. This usually takes five to six minutes. Make the first turn when they have formed a brown crust at the bottom but the dough on top is still runny, using a knitting needle or skewer.

4. Serve them hot with confectioner's sugar and your favorite jam.

HYGGE TIP: GET KNITTING

Why might someone have a knitting needle laying around? Because knitting is extremely hygge. It is a sign of "everything is safe"–it has a certain grandma vibe to it—and even the sound of knitting is hygge. Knitting also brings calmness to the situation and atmosphere. In fact, one of my friends is currently studying to be a midwife. She and her class were told by one of the professors that they should take up knitting because it would have a calming effect on people in the room when the babies were being delivered. Most of the students in the class were knitting during the next class. Oh, and of course, there are bonus hygge points for socks and scarves you've knitted yourself.

CHRISTMAS WOVEN HEARTS

There is a long tradition in Denmark for making pleated hearts out of paper as ornaments for the Christmas tree.

The origin of the tradition is unknown, but the oldest known heart was in fact made by Hans Christian Andersen in 1860. It is still kept in a museum. In the early twentieth century, making Christmas hearts became widespread, particularly perhaps because pleating the hearts out of glossy paper was considered to improve children's fine motor skills. Today families with kids will spend a healthy part of Sunday afternoons in December making Christmas hearts.

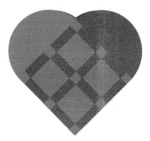

HOW TO MAKE WOVEN HEARTS

What you need: Two different-colored sheets of glossy paper (here, red and blue), a pair of scissors, a pencil, and a bit of patience.

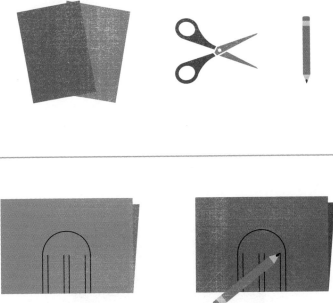

HEART X

HEART Y

STEP 1:

Fold the colored sheets of glossy paper in half. (If the paper is colored on only one side, make sure the colored side faces outward.)

On the outer side of each folded piece of paper, draw an outline of the U shape with 4 cut lines (one heart X and one heart Y). The straight edge of the U shape should be along the fold of the paper.

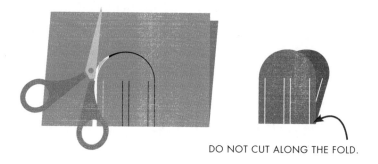

DO NOT CUT ALONG THE FOLD.

STEP 2:

Cut out the shapes including along the cut lines. You will have one cutout of each color.

Each cutout will have two layers of paper and five flaps.

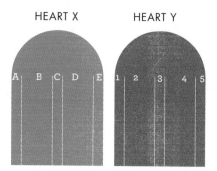

HEART X   HEART Y

A   B   C   D   E   1   2   3   4   5

STEP 3:

There are only two possible actions when pleating the flaps: a flap either goes through the middle of another flap or has another flap going through the middle of it. Adjacent flaps alternate, so if one flap goes through another, the adjacent flap will do the opposite.

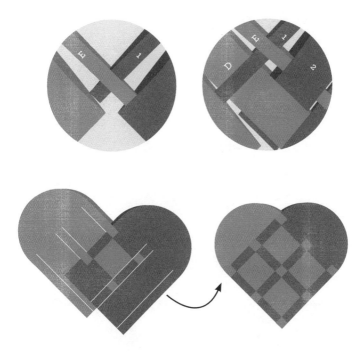

To create the woven heart, flap 1 of the blue cutout is threaded through the middle of flap E of the red cutout; flap D is threaded through flap 1; flap 1 through flap C; flap B through flap 1; and flap 1 through flap A.

Repeat this process starting with flap 2 but reverse the process beginning by threading flap E through flap 2.

Flap 3 must then be threaded like flap 1; flap 4 like flap 2; and flap 5 like flaps 3 and 1.

When flap 5 has been woven through flap A the heart is complete. You are now a qualified Dane!

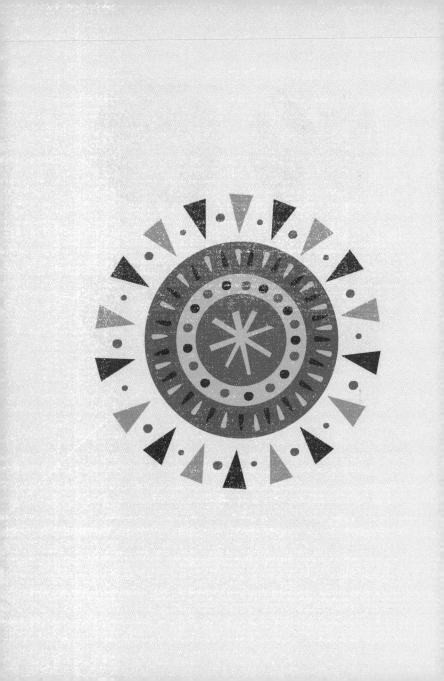

CHAPTER TWELVE

———

SUMMER HYGGE

THE LIVING IS EASY

———

While summer may not encourage the use of candles and fireplaces, summer can be hyggelig, *too. Summer is the smell of new-mown grass, suntanned skin, sunscreen, and salt water.*

It is reading in the shadow of a tree, enjoying the long summer nights, and standing around the barbecue with your friends. Summer doesn't mean you have to turn down the hygge. It is just a different kind of hygge from that of autumn or winter. It involves making use of the sun and the warmth and nature, but summer hygge still builds on the key elements of togetherness and good food. Here are five suggestions you can use to get the hygge going during summer.

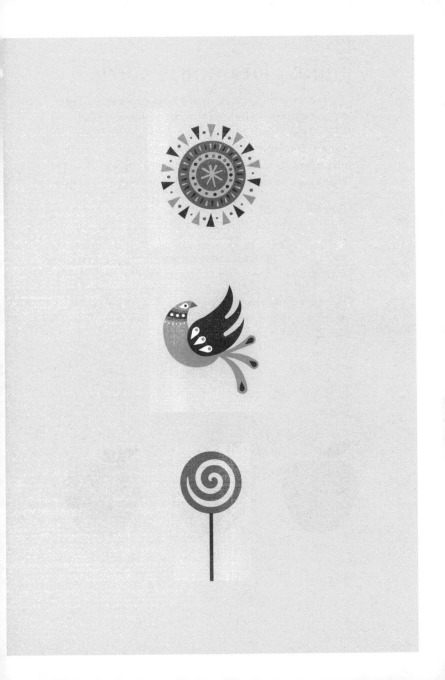

1. THINK CIDER HOUSE RULES

There are few things more *hyggelig* than spending a day in an orchard picking fruit. About once a year, my friends and I go to Fejø, a small island in the southern part of Denmark known for its apples. There are rows and rows of apple and plum trees. If we hit the island late in the summer, the Opal plums are ripe and the Filippa apples are ready.

Spending one day at the orchard allows you to hygge another day by making jams or preserving the fruit you picked in other ways. This year, I hope we can have a go at making cider. Maybe it's time for that pantry party we talked about earlier.

There are many pick-your-own farms scattered throughout the countryside in the UK, US, Canada, Australia, and New Zealand.

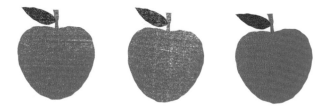

2. THROW A BARBECUE FOR FAMILY AND FRIENDS

Nothing gets the hygge going faster than lighting the barbecue. This is a type of hygge practiced in most parts of the world. Invite your friends and family over and get cooking together. Light the barbecue, and while you wait for the coals to get to just the right temperature, have a game of croquet.

3. JOIN OR BUILD A COMMUNITY GARDEN

At the moment, community gardens seem to be popping up everywhere, and with good reason. They are a wonderful way of getting the *hyggelig* atmosphere of a village into a bigger city. Tending to your tomatoes while having a chat with other gardeners is both *hyggelig* and meditative. In addition, it brings people in the local neighborhood together and fosters the development of community spirit. What's not to like?

Building community gardens was one of the proposals recommended by the Happiness Research Institute when we were working with a town just outside Copenhagen, trying to come up with ideas that would improve the social fabric and reduce isolation and loneliness in the community. But it was such a great idea that I thought we should build one ourselves. So we did. Across the street from our office is a church that has space for around twenty raised plant beds. We ordered seven tons of dirt and spent one Sunday afternoon building the garden, and of course, to top off the hygge, we finished the day with a barbecue.

4. PICNICS BY THE BEACH

Summer is a wonderful time of year to go to your local farmers' market and fill your basket with strawberries, cherries, and watermelon. Add some bread and cheese to the basket, and you're good to go. Bring all your friends, or just that one special person, and find a spot near the sea. This is the recipe for one of the most *hyggelig* activities you can do throughout the summer. A whole day can easily pass just in talking, reading, and enjoying the freedom of not having to do anything.

5. CARGO BIKE AROUND

What better way to experience your city or neighborhood than by cycling around it? Of course, being from Copenhagen, I might be biased in this regard. So if you have the good fortune—as I do—to know some good people who own a cargo bike, you might be able to borrow it for a day. A cargo bike is a bicycle that allows you to have a passenger or two. A three-wheeled bicycle with a large box in front for transporting your kids, your spouse, dog, groceries or whatever you want to take for a ride. Of course, you could walk or drive. But the cargo bike can be turned into a movable fortress of hygge.

Bring pillows, a blanket, treats, music, a picnic basket—whatever tickles your fancy. This is the perfect way to spend a summer afternoon, but if you add an extra warm blanket and a good sweater, this can also work as a year-round activity. In fact one winter, I biked a beautiful Swedish woman around under the Copenhagen Christmas lights in an attempt to woo her. The attempt failed. "The timing wasn't right" (which I believe translates into "I'm just not that into you" in every language), but I am sure it wasn't because she thought our date lacked hygge.

BIKES AND HAPPINESS

———

In addition to hygge, Hans Christian Andersen, Lego, and Danish design, Denmark is known for its love of bikes.

Of course, it is easy to be a nation of cyclophiliacs when the country's highest point is less than six hundred and fifty-six feet and when the city invests heavily in infrastructure for cyclists. (Car taxes of 150 to 180 percent probably also help.)

Nevertheless, Danes love their bikes and cycling. In Copenhagen, 45 percent of those who live, study, or work in the city cycle to their place of education or employment. Roughly a third of those working in the city but living outside it choose to commute by bicycle. I think most of us appreciate that cycling is an easy way to weave a bit of exercise into our daily routine and is environmentally (and wallet) friendly. However, that is not why Copenhageners bike. We do it because it is easy and convenient. It is simply the fastest way to get from A to B. But there is an additional advantage that may be overlooked and underappreciated: biking makes people happier.

A comprehensive study carried out in 2014 by researchers at the University of East Anglia's Norwich Medical School and the Center for Health Economics at the University of York, and based on nearly 18,000 adult commuters over eighteen years, found that people who bike to work are happier than those who drive or use public transport.

You might argue that we can't be sure that it's the cycling that causes the happiness. It could just as well be the other way round—

that the happier people are, the more inclined they are to cycle. True, but this is where it gets interesting. When the researchers of the study analyzed the results, they discovered that the people who over the years had changed from commuting by car or bus to cycling or going on foot became happier after the switch. And to further bombard you with compelling arguments to give the bike a try, another study, from McGill University in Montreal, also found that those who cycled to work were most satisfied with their commute, even though it could make their commute longer.

And if happiness isn't enough of a motivation, let me tell you that according to a Dutch (cyclophiliacs as well) study undertaken by the University of Utrecht, switching from driving to riding a bike in your daily commute adds three to fourteen months to your life expectancy, and a Danish study concluded—perhaps unsurprisingly—that children who cycled to school were significantly fitter than those who were driven.

"Okay," you might say. "So cycling will make me healthier and happier. But what good are health and happiness? They can't bring me money. . . " Well, you might not be the ideal target group for my next argument, but here goes: if you bike, we all win. It is good for the community.

Cycling is not only beneficial for the individual and his or her well-being and health, but it's an indicator of the degree of neighbors' and locals' sense of community. A Swedish study of 2012 of more than 21,000 people found that people who traveled by car generally attended fewer social events and family gatherings. Furthermore, the drivers had comparatively less trust in other people. Those who chose to walk or cycle to their destinations attended more social events and had a comparatively greater trust in others.

This doesn't mean that swapping your car for a bike will instantly improve how much you trust other people. The researchers behind the study point toward the increase in commuting distance as an explanation. Because of a more flexible and accessible labor market, people find jobs farther afield. In turn, this means that people's social networks are spread farther geographically, which reduces their sense of belonging and engagement in their neighborhood. In other words, if a city is designed in a way that makes a long drive to work necessary, we harm the social health of that city. If a lot of people cycle, it's probably an indication that you live in a healthy neighborhood. This is something that should be seriously considered in urban planning if we want to ensure neighborliness and trust among locals.

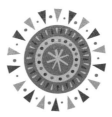

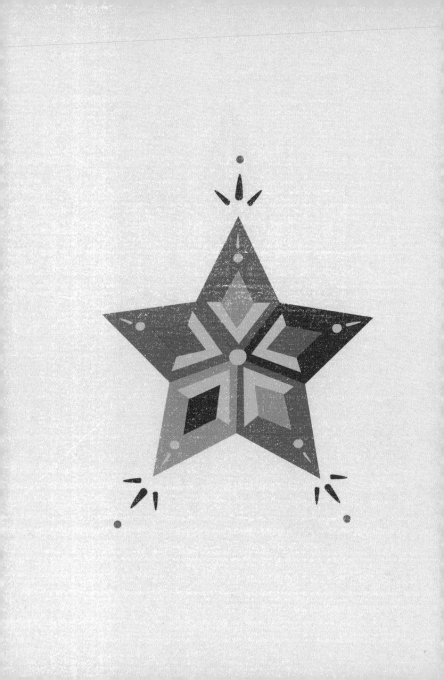

—

CHAPTER THIRTEEN

FIVE
DIMENSIONS
OF HYGGE

While hygge can be an intangible and abstract concept, I do believe that we can use all our senses to detect it. Hygge has a taste, a sound, a smell and a texture—and, hopefully, you will start to see hygge all around.

THE TASTE OF HYGGE

Taste is an important element of hygge because it often involves eating something. And that something cannot be too fresh, alternative or challenging in any way.

The taste of hygge is almost always familiar, sweet, and comforting. If you want to make a cup of tea more *hyggelig*, you add honey. If you want to make a cake more *hyggelig*, you add icing. And if you want your stew to be more *hyggelig*, you add wine.

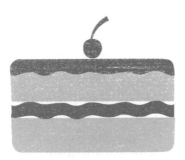

THE SOUND OF HYGGE

The small sparks and dynamic crackles of burning wood are probably the most hyggelige *sounds there are. But don't worry if you live in an apartment and cannot have an open fire without also facing great risk of death.*

Many sounds can be *hyggelige*. Actually, hygge mainly has to do with the absence of sounds, which enables you to hear even very quiet noises such as raindrops on the roof, wind blowing outside the window, the sound of trees waving in the wind, or the creaks of wooden planks that yield when you walk on them. Also, the sounds of a person drawing, cooking, or knitting could be *hyggelig*. Any sound of a safe environment will be the soundtrack of hygge. For example, the sound of thunder can be very *hyggeligt* if you are inside and feel safe; if outside, not so much.

SMELLS LIKE HYYGE

Have you ever smelled something that takes you back to a time and place where you felt safe? Or smelled something that, more than a memory, gives you a flashback of how the world used to look when you were a child?

Or maybe the smell of something provokes strong feelings of security and comfort, such as the aroma coming from a bakery, or the smell of apple trees in your childhood garden or maybe the familiar scent of your parents' house?

What makes a smell *hyggelig* differs very much from person to person, because smells relate a situation to ones experienced with that smell in the past. For some people, the smell of cigarettes in the morning is the most *hyggelig* thing there is; to others, the smell may provoke nausea and headaches. One common element of all the smells of hygge is that they remind us of safety and the sense of being cared for. We use smell to sense whether something is safe to eat, but we also use it to intuit whether a place is safe and how alert we should be. The smell of hygge is the smell that tells you to put your guard down completely. The smell of cooking, the smell of a blanket you use at home, or the smell of a place we perceive as safe can be very *hyggeligt* because it reminds us of a state of mind we experienced when we felt completely safe.

WHAT DOES HYGGE FEEL LIKE?

As I mentioned earlier, letting your fingers run across a wooden surface, around a warm ceramic cup, or through the hairs on the skin of a reindeer brings out the hygge.

Old, homemade stuff that has taken a lot of time to make is always more *hyggeligt* than manufactured new stuff. And small things are always more *hyggeligt* than big things. If the slogan for the USA is "The bigger, the better," the slogan for Denmark is "The smaller, the more *hyggeligt*."

In Copenhagen, almost all the buildings stand only three or four stories high. New houses made out of concrete, glass, and steel do not stand a chance against the hygge factor in these old buildings. Anything hand-crafted—objects created out of wood, ceramics, wool, leather, and so on—is *hyggeligt*. Shiny metal and glass are not *hyggeligt*—though they can be if they are old enough. The rustic, organic surface of something imperfect or something that has been or will be affected by age appeals to the touch of hygge. Also, the feeling of being inside something warm in a place where it is cold is very different from just being warm. It gives the feeling of being comfortable in a hostile environment.

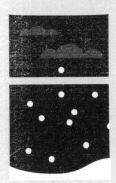

SEEING HYGGE

---

*Hygge is very much about light, as we have said.
Too bright is not* hyggeligt. *But hygge is also
very much about taking your time.*

This can be accentuated by watching very slow movements of
things, for example, gently falling snow—or *aqilokoq*, as the Inuits
would say—or the lazy flames from an open fire. In short, slow,
organic movements and dark, natural colors are *hyggelige*. The
sight of a bright, sterile hospital or watching fast-moving vehicles
on a highway is not. Hygge is dimmed, rustic, and slow.

THE SIXTH SENSE
OF HYGGE

―――――――――

Hygge is about feeling safe. Hence, hygge is an indication that you trust the ones you are with and where you are.

And the feeling of hygge is an indication of your feeling of pleasure when someone tells you to go with your gut feeling, that you have expanded your comfort zone to include other people and feel you can be completely yourself around other people.

So hygge can be tasted, heard, smelled, touched and seen. But, most important, hygge is felt. In the beginning of the book, I mentioned Winnie-the-Pooh, and I think his wisdom still holds true. You don't spell love. You feel it. This brings us to the final theme of the book: happiness.

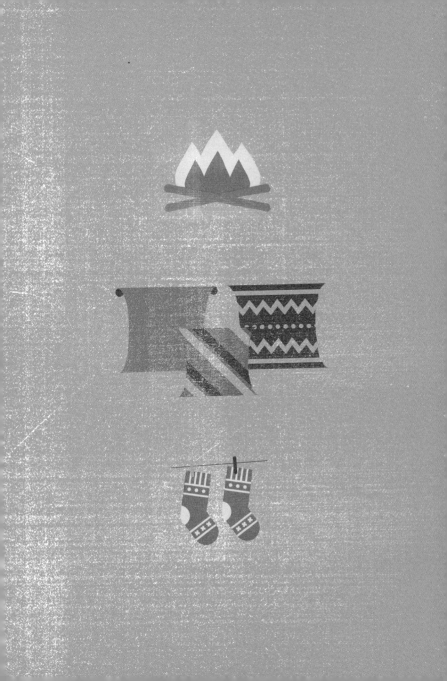

—

CHAPTER FOURTEEN

HYGGE AND HAPPINESS

Today, political leaders from around the world are expressing an interest in why some societies are happier than others. At the same time, countries are taking steps to measure their success as a society—not only from how much the economy grows, but also from how much their lives are improved, not just by the standard of living but quality of life. This is one of the consequences of the paradigm shift away from gross domestic product (GDP) as the dominant indicator for progress in recent years. However, this idea is not new. As Robert Kennedy pointed out more than forty years ago:

> *The gross national product does not allow for the health of our children, the quality of their education or the joy of their play. It does not include the beauty of our poetry or the strength of our marriages; the intelligence of our public debate or the integrity of our public officials ... it measures everything, in short, except that which makes life worthwhile.*

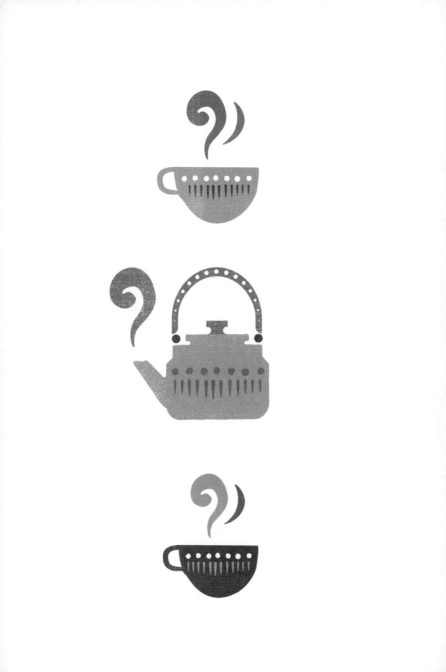

Lately, this has increased the interest in and number of happiness surveys—and it seems that Denmark comes out on top almost every time. "About once a year, some new study confirms Denmark's status as a happiness superpower," wrote a journalist at *The New York Times* in 2009. Since then, the statement has become even truer.

The World Happiness Report, which is commissioned by the United Nations, has now been published four times. Denmark has been in first place every time except once, when the country was pushed to third place. And the World Happiness Report is just one out of many rankings that puts Denmark and Copenhagen at the top of the lists about happiness and the country's livability.

The same pattern is evident when the Organization for Economic Co-operation and Development looks at life satisfaction and when the European Social Survey looks at happiness. *Monocle* magazine has several times ranked Copenhagen as the world's most livable city. Nowadays, well-being rankings are only news in Denmark when the country doesn't make first place. In addition, most Danes can't help but smile a little when they hear that Denmark is the happiest country in the world. They are well aware that Denmark was not first in line when weather was handed out and that when they are sitting in traffic on a wet February morning, they hardly look like the world's happiest people.

So why are the people in Denmark so happy?

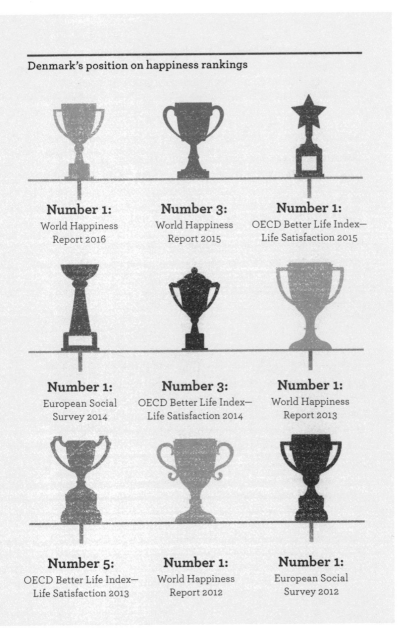

Denmark's position on happiness rankings

Number 1:
World Happiness
Report 2016

Number 3:
World Happiness
Report 2015

Number 1:
OECD Better Life Index—
Life Satisfaction 2015

Number 1:
European Social
Survey 2014

Number 3:
OECD Better Life Index—
Life Satisfaction 2014

Number 1:
World Happiness
Report 2013

Number 5:
OECD Better Life Index—
Life Satisfaction 2013

Number 1:
World Happiness
Report 2012

Number 1:
European Social
Survey 2012

THE HAPPY DANES

As discussed, international surveys frequently name Denmark as the happiest country in the world, and this has naturally prompted an increasing interest on the part of happiness researchers. What are the reasons behind the high levels of happiness in Denmark?

At the Happiness Research Institute, we have tried to answer this question in the report "The Happy Danes—Exploring the Reasons for the High Level of Happiness in Denmark." Briefly, there are many reasons. Several factors influence why some people and countries are happier than others:—genetics, our relationships, health, income, job, sense of purpose and freedom.

But one of the main reasons why Denmark does so well in international happiness surveys is the welfare state, as it reduces uncertainty, worries, and stress in the population. You can say that Denmark is the happiest country in the world or you can say that Denmark is the least unhappy country in the world. The welfare state is really good (not perfect, but good) at reducing extreme unhappiness. Universal and free health care, free university education, and relatively generous unemployment benefits go a long way toward reducing unhappiness. This has particular significance for those who are less well off, a segment of society who is happier in Denmark than in other wealthy countries.

Furthermore, there is a high level of trust in Denmark (notice all the strollers parked outside cafés when the parents are inside, drinking coffee). There is a high level of freedom (Danes report really high levels in terms of feeling in control over their lives), of wealth and good governance, and a well-functioning civil society.

These factors, however, don't set Denmark apart from other Nordic countries. Norway, Sweden, Finland, and Iceland also enjoy relatively high levels of welfare. This is why all the Nordic countries are usually found in the top ten of happiness rankings. However, maybe the instance of hygge is what sets Denmark apart from the rest of the Nordic countries. I think hygge and happiness might be linked, as hygge may be the pursuit of everyday happiness and some of the key components of hygge are drivers of happiness. Let's look at some of them.

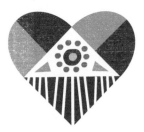

HYGGE AS
SOCIAL SUPPORT

Given the above, we can now perhaps explain three-quarters of the reasons why some countries are happier than others—factors such as generosity, freedom, GDP, good governance, and healthy life expectancy. But the factor that has the biggest effect on our happiness is social support.

What is meant by this is simply: do people have someone in their network they can rely on in times of need? Yes or no. It might not be the best or most nuanced way of measuring our social support systems, but it is the data we have across as many countries as are covered by the World Happiness Report.

One of the reasons for the high level of happiness in Denmark is the good work–life balance, which allows people to make time for family and friends. According to the OECD Better Life Index, Danes have more free time than all the other OECD members, and according to the European Social Survey, 33 percent of Danes report feeling calm and peaceful all or most of the time, while the percentages are 23 for Germany, 15 in France, and 14 in the United Kingdom.

So policies matter, but maybe hygge also fosters a special way of being together with your loved ones. In the chapter on togetherness, we touched on the link between relationships, hygge, and happiness.

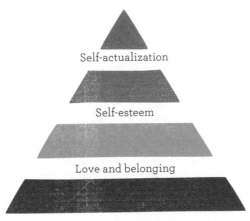

Self-actualization

Self-esteem

Love and belonging

Food, water, sleep, and security

This link cannot be overstated. In 1943, the American psychologist Abraham Maslow developed a model called the pyramid of human needs and the theory that we must fill our needs from the bottom of the pyramid upward. The most elementary needs are physiological: food, water, and sleep—and security. But then come our social needs, our need for love and belonging. Without having these needs covered, we will not be able to move on to fulfilling our needs for self-esteem and self-actualization.

Today, when happiness researchers analyze the common denominators among those who consider themselves happy, a pattern emerges without exception: happy people have meaningful and positive social relationships. Studies also show that when individuals experience social isolation, many of the same brain regions become active that are active in the experience of physical pain.

The four editions of the World Happiness Report published thus far are packed with evidence of the link between relationships and happiness. Family and friends and close personal relationships with loved adults explain the greatest variation in happiness. Except in the very poorest countries, happiness varies more with the quality of our relationships than with wealth.

According to the reports, the most important relationships are with loved ones—across all societies—but our relationships at work, with friends, and in the community are also important. So quality relationships impact our happiness, but the causality goes both ways. Studies suggest that having high levels of happiness leads to better social relationships. The reason may be that happiness increases our level of sociability and improves the quality of the relationships we have. Experiments also show that people in a positive mood express greater interest in social and pro-social activities. Similarly, according to the World Happiness Report, a world survey of 123 nations found that the experience of positive feelings was strongly related to good social relationships across different sociocultural regions.

In sum, research from several decades provides evidence that supports the bond between our relationships and well-being. Happier people have a larger quantity and better quality of friendships and family relationships. Thus good relationships both cause happiness and are caused by it. The studies suggest that, of all the factors that influence happiness, a sense of feeling related to those around you is very near the top of the list.

This is why hygge may be one of the reasons that Danes always report high levels of happiness. Not only are there policies that secure them time to pursue meaningful relationships, but the language and the culture also drive Danes to prioritize spending time with family and friends and to develop quality relationships over time.

SAVORING AND GRATITUDE

As mentioned in the chapter on food, hygge is about giving yourself and others a treat. It is about savoring the moment and the simple pleasures of good food and good company.

It is giving the hot chocolate with whipped cream the attention it deserves. In short, indulgence. Hygge is about the *now*, how to enjoy the moment and make the best of it.

More than anything, savoring is about gratitude. We often remind each other not to take things for granted. Gratitude is more than just a simple "thank you" when you receive a gift. It is about keeping in mind that you live right now, allowing yourself to focus on the moment and appreciate the life you lead, to focus on all that you do have, not what you don't. Clichés? Totally.

Nevertheless, evidence-based studies show that practicing gratitude has an impact on happiness.

According to Robert A. Emmons, a professor of psychology at University of California, Davis, and one of the world's leading experts on gratitude, people who feel grateful are not only happier than those who do not but also more helpful and forgiving and less materialistic.

In one of his studies, which involved interviewing over a thousand people, some were told to keep gratitude journals, writing down what they were grateful for on a weekly basis. The researchers found that gratitude has psychological, physical, and social benefits. The people who wrote the gratitude journals reported feeling more positive emotions like alertness and enthusiasm, reported better sleep and fewer symptoms of disease, and were more mindful of situations where they could be helpful.

Research also shows that grateful people tend to recover more quickly from trauma and suffering than others and are less likely to get stressed in different situations. You can see why it is important to include gratitude in your everyday life.

Unfortunately, since our emotional system is a fan of newness, we are quick to adapt to new things and events, especially positive ones. Therefore, you need to come up with new things to be grateful for, and not get stuck in the same way of thinking. Emmons believes that gratitude makes people take a step back and see the value of what they have and thereby appreciate it more, which makes it less likely that they will take it for granted.

Hygge may help us to be grateful for the everyday because it is all about savoring simple pleasures. Hygge is making the most of the moment, but hygge is also a way of planning for and preserving happiness. Danes plan for *hyggelige* times and reminisce about them afterward.

"Is nostalgia part of hygge?" one of the designers of this book asked me. He had read some of the first drafts and we were now discussing the feel and visual identity at the Granola Café at Værnedamsvej in Copenhagen. At first I dismissed his idea. But in the process of writing, I slowly realized that he was right. Reliving hygge moments, sitting in front of the fire or on a balcony in the French Alps, or walking back into the summer cabin of my childhood, I was tripping on nostalgia. At the same time, I noticed that I was smiling.

According to the study "Nostalgia: Content, Triggers, Function" in the *Journal of Personality and Social Psychology* (November 2006), nostalgia produces positive feelings, reinforces our memories and sense of being loved, and boosts self-esteem. So while happiness and hygge are definitely about appreciating the now, both may also be planned and preserved. Hygge and happiness have a past and a future as well as a present.

HYGGE AS EVERYDAY HAPPINESS

———

I study happiness. Each day, I try to answer one question: why are some people happier than others?

I've been told that musicians can look at notes and hear the music in their heads. The same thing happens to me when I look at happiness data. I hear comforting sounds of lives well lived. I hear the joy, the feeling of connectedness, and the sense of purpose.

Many people are, however, skeptical about the possibility of measuring happiness. One of the issues raised is that there are different perceptions of what happiness is. We try to acknowledge this by saying that "happiness" is an umbrella term. We break it down and look at the different components. So when the Happiness Research Institute, the UN, the OECD, and different governments try to measure happiness and quantify quality of life, we can consider at least three dimensions of happiness.

First of all, we look at life satisfaction. We do this by asking people in international surveys: How satisfied are you with your life all in all? Or how happy are you on a scale from 0 to 10? Take a step back and evaluate your life. Think of the best possible life you could lead and the worst possible: Where do you feel you stand right now? This is where Denmark scores the highest in the world.

Second, we look at the affective or hedonic dimension. What kind of emotions do people experience on an everyday basis? If you look at yesterday, did you feel angry, sad, lonely? Did you laugh? Did you feel happy? Did you feel loved?

The third dimension is called the eudaemonic dimension. That is named after the ancient Greek word *eudaimonia* for "happiness." And it is based on Aristotle's perception of happiness. To him, the good life was a meaningful life. So do people experience a sense of purpose?

Ideally, what we do is follow ten thousand or more people—in a scientific manner, not like a stalker—over, say, ten years. Because, over the next decade, some of us are going to get a promotion, some of us are going to lose our job, and some of us are going to get married. The question is: How do those changes in life circumstances impact the different dimensions of happiness?

So how happy are you all in all? How satisfied are you with your life? These questions have been asked and answered millions of times across the world, so now we can look for patterns in the data. What do happy people have in common, whether you are from Denmark, the UK, the US, China, or India? What is the average effect on happiness from, say, doubling your income or getting married? What are the common denominators of happiness?

We have been doing this for years when it comes to health, for example, looking into the common denominators of people who live to be a hundred years old. And because of those studies, we know that alcohol, tobacco, exercise, and our diet have an effect on our life expectancy. We use the same methods to understand what matters for happiness.

So you might say, "Well, happiness is very subjective." Yes, of course it is, and it should be. What I care about is how you feel about your life. I think you are the best judge of whether you are happy or not. Yes, working with subjective measures is difficult, but it is not impossible. We do it all the time when it comes to stress, anxiety, and depression, which are also in some senses subjective phenomena. At the end of the day, it is all about how we as individuals perceive our lives. I have yet to hear a convincing argument why happiness should be the one thing in the world we cannot study in a scientific manner. Why should we not try to understand the thing that perhaps matters the most?

So we try to understand what drives life satisfaction, affective or hedonic happiness, and eudaemonia. The different dimensions are linked, of course. If you have a day-to-day life that is filled with positive emotions, you are likely to report higher levels of life satisfaction. But the second dimension is much more volatile. We can detect a weekend effect here. People report more positive emotions during weekends than on weekdays. This would come as no surprise to most people, as we are more likely to engage in activities that bring out positive emotions during the weekend. Furthermore, the different dimensions of happiness are linked biologically. For instance, hedonic and eudaemonic well-being are correlated, and many of the brain mechanisms involved in the hedonic experience of sensory pleasure are also active in the more eudaemonic experience.

Coming back to hygge and happiness, I think that one of the most interesting findings in recent years is that the experience of positive emotions matters more to our overall well-being, measured in terms of life satisfaction, than the absence of negative emotions (although both are important, according to the World Happiness Report).

Researching and writing this book, I have come to realize that hygge may function as a driver for happiness on an everyday basis. Hygge gives us the language, the objective, and the methods for planning and preserving happiness—and for getting a little bit of it every day. Hygge may be the closest we come to happiness when we arrive home after a long day's work on a cold, rainy day in January.

And let's face it, this is where most of our lives will play out. Not on cold, January days, but every day. Once a year—or more, if we are lucky—we may find ourselves on a beach in some exotic country and we may find both hygge and happiness on these distant shores. But hygge is about making the most of what we have in abundance: the everyday. Perhaps Benjamin Franklin said it best: "Happiness consists more in small conveniences or pleasures that occur every day, than in great pieces of good fortune that happen but seldom."

Now, I am off to see my dad and his wife. I think I will take cake.

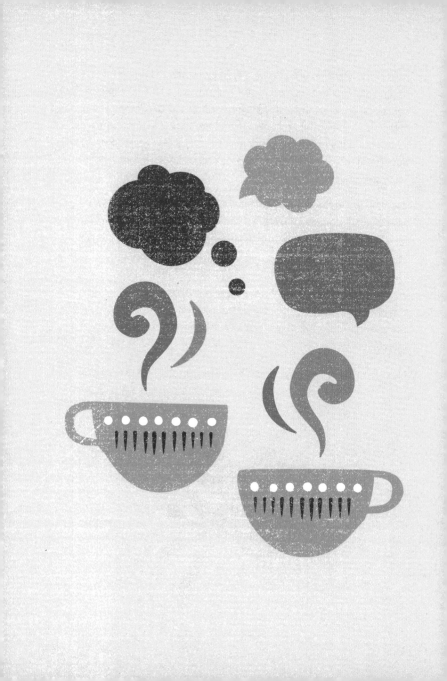

ACKNOWLEDGMENTS

I would like to thank the researchers at the Happiness Research Institute—Johan, Felicia, Michael, and Kjartan—for their help with this book. Without them, work would not be half as hyggeligt.

La Glace, June 2016

ABOUT THE AUTHOR

Meik Wiking is CEO of the Happiness Research Institute, research associate for Denmark at the World Database of Happiness, and founding member of the Latin American Network for Wellbeing and Quality of Life Policies. He and his research have been featured in more than five hundred media outlets, including *The Washington Post*, BBC, *Huffington Post*, the *Times* (London), *The Guardian*, CBS, Monocle, the *Atlantic*, and PBS News Hour. He has spoken at TEDx, and his books have been translated into more than fifteen languages. He lives in Copenhagen, Denmark.

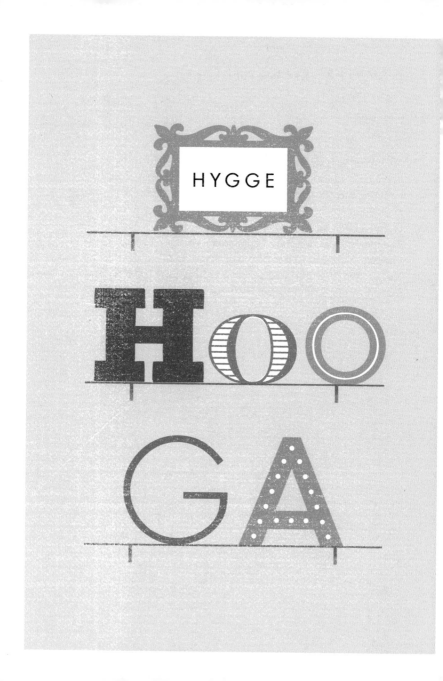